POCKET GUIDE TO

Bariatric Surgery

THIRD EDITION

Weight Management Dietetic Practice Group

Editors

Kellene A. Isom
PhD, MS, RD, CAGS

Melissa C. Majumdar
MS, RD, CSOWM, LDN

Academy of Nutrition and Dietetics
Chicago, IL

eat right. Academy of Nutrition and Dietetics

Academy of Nutrition and Dietetics
120 S. Riverside Plaza, Suite 2190
Chicago, IL 60606

Academy of Nutrition and Dietetics Pocket Guide to Bariatric Surgery, Third Edition

ISBN 978-0-88091-191-7 (print)
ISBN 978-0-88091-208-2 (eBook)
Catalog Number 424622 (print)
Catalog Number 424622e (eBook)

10 9 8 7 6 5 4 3 2 1

For more information on the Academy of Nutrition and Dietetics, visit www.eatright.org.

Library of Congress Cataloging-in-Publication Data

Names: Isom, Kellene A., editor. | Majumdar, Melissa (Melissa C.), editor. | American Dietetic Association. Weight Management Dietetic Practice Group, editor.
Title: Pocket guide to bariatric surgery / Weight Management Dietetic Practice Gro ; editors, Kellene A. Isom, PhD, MS, RD, CAGS, Melissa C. Majumdar, MS, RD, CSOWM, LDN.
Other titles: Academy of Nutrition and Dietetics pocket guide to bariatric surgery.
Description: Third edition. | Chicago, IL : Academy of Nutrition and Dietetics, [2022] | Preceded by: Academy of Nutrition and Dietetics pocket guide to bariatric surgery / Weight Management Dietetic Practice Group ; Sue Cummings and Kellene A. Isom, editors, 2015. Second edition. | Includes bibliographical references and index.
Identifiers: LCCN 2021030435 (print) | LCCN 2021030436 (ebook) | ISBN 9780880911917 (spiral bound) | ISBN 9780880912082 (ebook)
Subjects: LCSH: Obesity--Surgery--Handbooks, manuals, etc.
Classification: LCC RD540 .A26 2022 (print) | LCC RD540 (ebook) | DDC 617.4/3--dc23
LC record available at https://lccn.loc.gov/2021030435
LC ebook record available at https://lccn.loc.gov/2021030436

Contents

List of Boxes, Tables, and Figures

Boxes

Tables

Figures

Frequently Used Terms and Abbreviations

AACE	American Association of Clinical Endocrinologists
AAP	American Academy of Pediatrics
ACS	American College of Surgeons
AGB	adjustable gastric band
ASA	American Society of Anesthesiologists
ASMBS	American Society for Metabolic and Bariatric Surgery
ASPEN	American Society for Parenteral and Enteral Nutrition
BMI	body mass index
BMR	basal metabolic rate
BOLD	Bariatric Outcomes Longitudinal Database
BP	biliopancreatic
BPD	biliopancreatic diversion
BPD/DS	biliopancreatic diversion with duodenal switch
BUN	blood urea nitrogen
CBC	complete blood count
CBT	cognitive behavioral therapy

CDC	Centers for Disease Control and Prevention
CKD	chronic kidney disease
CSOWM	Certified Specialist in Obesity and Weight Management
DEXA	dual-energy x-ray absorptiometry
DFE	dietary folate equivalent
DIAAS	Digestible Indispensable Amino Acid Score
DPG	dietetic practice group
EAL	Academy of Nutrition and Dietetics Evidence Analysis Library
EBT	Endoscopic Bariatric Therapies
EBW	excess body weight
EN	enteral nutrition
ESG	endoscopic sleeve gastroplasty
EWL	excess weight loss
FDA	Food and Drug Administration
FFM	fat-free mass
GDM	gestational diabetes mellitus
GERD	gastroesophageal reflux disease
GI	gastrointestinal
GLP-1	glucagon-like peptide 1
H&P	history and physical
HbA1c	hemoglobin A1c
HDL	high-density lipoprotein
IAA	indispensable amino acids
IBW	ideal body weight
IFSO	International Federation for the Surgery of Obesity

IGB	intragastric balloons
iPTH	intact parathyroid hormone
IV	intravenous
LOC	loss of control
LOS	length of stay
MBS	metabolic and bariatric surgery
MBSAQIP	Metabolic and Bariatric Surgery Accreditation and Quality Improvement Program
MGB	mini-gastric bypass
MI	motivational interviewing
MMA	methylmalonic acid
MNT	medical nutrition therapy
NASH	nonalcoholic steatohepatitis
NCP	Nutrition Care Process
NHLBI	National Heart, Lung, and Blood Institute
NIDDKD	National Institute of Diabetes and Digestive and Kidney Diseases
NIH	National Institutes of Health
NSV	nonscale victory
OAC	Obesity Action Coalition
OAGB	one-anastomosis gastric bypass
ODS	Office of Dietary Supplements
OHS	obesity hypoventilation syndrome
OMA	Obesity Medicine Association
OTC	over-the-counter
PBH	postbariatric hypoglycemia

PCP	primary care provider
PDCAAS	protein digestibility-corrected amino acid score
%EBMIL	percent excess body mass index loss
%EWL	percentage of excess weight loss
%TBWL	percentage of total body weight loss
%TWL	percentage of total weight loss
PES	problem, etiology, and symptoms
PN	parenteral nutrition
POD	postoperative day
POSE	Primary obesity surgery endoluminal
PPI	proton pump inhibitor
PSU	Penn State University
PYY	peptide YY
RAE	retinol activity equivalent
RCT	randomized controlled trial
RDN	registered dietitian nutritionist
RMR	resting metabolic rate
RYGB	Roux-en-Y gastric bypass
SADI-S	single-anastomosis duodeno-ileostomy with sleeve
SG	sleeve gastrectomy
SGA	small for gestational age
SIBO	small intestinal bacteria overgrowth
T2DM	type 2 diabetes mellitus
TBWL	total body weight loss
TIBC	total iron-binding capacity
TOS	The Obesity Society

TTM	transtheoretical model
TWL	total weight loss
UGI	upper gastrointestinal series
UL	tolerable upper limit
WM	weight management
WNL	within normal limits

Contributors

Editors

Kellene A. Isom, PhD, MS, RD, CAGS
Assistant Professor, Nutrition, California State Polytechnic University, Pomona
Pomona, CA

Melissa C. Majumdar, MS, RD, CSOWM, LDN
Bariatric Coordinator, Emory University Hospital Midtown
Atlanta, GA

Authors

Laura Andromalos, MS, RD, CSOWM, CDCES
Clinical Nutrition Manager, University of Minnesota Medical Center—Sodexo
Minneapolis, MN

Katie Chapmon, MS, RD
Private Practice Dietitian and Speaker
Los Angeles, CA

Lillian Craggs-Dino, DHA, RDN, LDN
Bariatric Dietitian and Support Group Coordinator, Cleveland Clinic Florida
Weston, FL

Mary Gray Hixson, MPH, RD, CSOWM, LDN
Bariatric Nutrition Supervisor and Lead Dietitian, North Carolina Surgery-Rex Bariatrics, University North Carolina REX Healthcare
Raleigh, NC

Kellene A. Isom, PhD, MS, RD, CAGS
Assistant Professor, Nutrition, California State Polytechnic University, Pomona
Pomona, CA

Abigail Holewinski, MS, RD
Clinical Research Manager, GID Bio, Inc
Louisville, CO

Heather K. Mackie, MS, RD, LD
Clinical Director, ReShape Lifesciences, Inc
Montgomery, TX

Melissa C. Majumdar, MS, RD, CSOWM, LDN
Bariatric Coordinator, Emory University Hospital Midtown
Atlanta, GA

Kris M. Mogensen, MS, RD-AP, LDN, CNSC
Team Leader Dietitian Specialist, Department of Nutrition, Brigham and Women's Hospital
Boston, MA

Frances Parpos, RD, LDN, CDCES
Senior Nutritionist, Cardiac Rehabilitation, Brigham and Women's Hospital
Foxborough, MA

Susan Sewell, MS, RD, CSOWM, LD
Registered Dietitian, Diabetes Educator,
Cincinnati Children's Hospital
Cincinnati, OH

Cassie I. Story, RDN
Private Practice Dietitian, WLS Daily, Director of Nutrition Education, Bariatric Advantage
Scottsdale, AZ

Colleen Tewksbury, PhD, MPH, RD, CSOWM, LDN
Senior Research Investigator, Perelman School of Medicine, University of Pennsylvania
Philadelphia, PA

Reviewers

Laura Andromalos, MS, RD, CSOWM, CDCES
Clinical Nutrition Manager, University of Minnesota Medical Center—Sodexo
Minneapolis, MN

Svetlana Chentsova, FNP-BC, RN-BC, CBN
Nurse Practitioner Team Manager, Brigham and Women's Hospital
Boston, MA

Nina Crowley, PhD, RDN, LD
Metabolic & Bariatric Surgery Program Coordinator, Medical University of South Carolina
Charleston, SC

Liz Goldenberg, MPH, RD, CDN
Bariatric Surgery Program Coordinator, Weill Cornell Medicine, New York Presbyterian Hospital
New York, NY

Molly Jones Mills, RDN, LD
Outpatient Bariatric Surgery Dietitian and Adolescent Program Coordinator, Sodexo/The Medical University of South Carolina
Charleston, SC

Kristen Smith, MS, RDN, LD
Bariatric Surgery Program Coordinator, Piedmont Atlanta Hospital
Atlanta, GA

Preface

In the 6 short years since the second edition of the *Academy of Nutrition and Dietetics Pocket Guide to Bariatric Surgery* was published, the metabolic and bariatric surgery (MBS) literature has exploded. The sleeve gastrectomy has officially become the most performed surgery, and the popularity of endoscopic procedures has increased. The third edition of the *Academy of Nutrition and Dietetics Pocket Guide to Bariatric Surgery* is meant to serve as a snapshot into the most up-to-date literature to support the registered dietitian nutritionist (RDN) and the interdisciplinary team to care for the MBS patient with evidence-based practices. The RDN new to MBS practice may use the pocket guide to gather background on the medical and nutrition components of MBS surgery, or the RDN who has devoted their career to the care of the MBS patient may refer to this book to validate the care of the complex patient with kidney disease, pregnancy, or nutritional deficiencies.

The third edition includes updates to reflect the gains in the literature and shifts in the field:

- Descriptions of single anastomosis procedures have been added to Chapter 1.
- More long-term data on the outcomes of MBS have been added.
- The biliopancreatic diversion with duodenal switch is included throughout the pocket guide.
- More liberal diet progression options are reviewed in Chapter 3 and Appendix B.
- Nutrition-related enhanced recovery interventions are discussed in Chapters 2 and 3.

- A more thorough review of MBS in adolescents is included in Chapter 6, as practitioners and researchers now have more studies in the adolescent population.
- A full chapter (Chapter 9) is devoted to endoscopic weight loss therapies: balloons, aspiration therapies, and revisional procedures performed endoscopically.
- Appendixes C and D, which deal with vitamin and mineral supplementation and biochemical surveillance, have been reformatted. They now include easy-to-interpret tables with valuable updates for the treatment of nutritional deficiencies in the MBS patient.
- A new appendix on nutrition counseling and education (Appendix H) has been added to relate evidence-based counseling methods and theories of change to the MBS population.

Acknowledgments

We would like to thank the authors and reviewers for their perseverance during a global pandemic and devotion to evidence-based practice. We appreciate the thorough and careful feedback of our peer reviewers. It is with the teamwork and attention to detail of this esteemed group that we can produce this valuable resource.

We would like to acknowledge Sue Cummings, MS, RD, LDN, for providing the foundation for this work in the first and second editions of the text. We would also like to thank Mary Litchford, PhD, RDN, LDN, for her intellect on protein quality (Chapter 3) and Edo Aarts, MD, PhD, for his surgical drawings (Chapter 1). We also appreciate the support and patience of our family and friends, as we have edited during late nights and weekend mornings.

Publisher's Note on Gender-Inclusive Language

The Academy of Nutrition and Dietetics encourages diversity and inclusion by striving to recognize, respect, and include differences in ability, age, creed, culture, ethnicity, gender, gender identity, political affiliation, race, religion, sexual orientation, size, and socioeconomic characteristics in the nutrition and dietetics profession.[1]

As part of our commitment to diversity and inclusion, all new and updated editions of professional books and practitioner resources published by the Academy of Nutrition and Dietetics will transition to the use of inclusive language. As appropriate, gender-neutral language, such as person/persons, individual/individuals, or patient/patients, is used to respect and recognize the spectrum of gender identities, including transgender and nonbinary identities. Where gender or sex is referred to in this book, it is important to note that data on sex assigned at birth or gender identity were not further specified for study participants, and specific recommendations or data for transgender and gender-diverse-people were not provided.

Existing guidelines for nutrition assessment and interventions rely primarily on gender-specific values and recommendations. As research continues to explore the unique health and nutrition needs of transgender and gender-diverse people, nutrition and health practitioners can expand their knowledge and understanding by reviewing available resources that provide general guidance for person-centered nutrition care of gender-diverse individuals.[2-4] The use of inclusive language is consistent with the American Medical Association's *AMA Manual of Style*[5] as well as other health professional groups and government organizations. The Academy of Nutrition and Dietetics will continue to evolve to adopt consensus best practices related to nutrition care of gender-diverse individuals that maximize inclusivity and improve equitable and evidence-based care.

1. Diversity and Inclusion Statement. Academy of Nutrition and Dietetics website. Accessed July 16, 2021. www.eatrightpro.org/practice/practice-resources/diversity-and-inclusion
2. Rozga M, Linsenmeyer W, Cantwell Wood J, Darst V, Gradwell EK. Hormone therapy, health outcomes and the role of nutrition in transgender individuals: A scoping review. *Clinical Nutrition ESPEN*. 2020;40:42-56. doi:10.1016/j.clnesp.2020.08.011
3. Rahman R, Linsenmeyer WR. Caring for transgender patients and clients: nutrition-related clinical and psychosocial considerations. *J Acad Nutr Diet*. 2019;119(5):727-732. doi:10.1016/j.jand.2018.03.006CTICE
4. Fergusson P, Greenspan N, Maitland L, Huberdeau R. Towards providing culturally aware nutritional care for transgender people: key issues and considerations. *Can J Diet Pract Res*. 2018;79(2):74-79. doi: 0.3148/cjdpr-2018-001.
5. JAMA Network. *AMA Manual of Style*. 11th ed. Oxford University Press; 2020; 543-544.

CHAPTER 1

Overview of Metabolic and Bariatric Surgery

Introduction

From 2017 to 2018, 42.4% and 9.2% of US adults met the criteria for obesity and severe obesity, respectively. The trends are unfortunately similar for children and adolescents in the United States. From 2015 to 2016, 18.5% of US adults met the criteria for obesity. The prevalence of both obesity and clinically severe obesity was highest in non-Hispanic Black adults compared to other races and Hispanic-origin groups. Adults aged 40 to 59 years were more likely to suffer from clinically severe obesity compared with other age groups.[1,2]

The increase in clinically severe obesity among adults in the United States continues to fuel the demand for metabolic and bariatric surgery (MBS). Approximately 252,000 MBS procedures were performed in the United States in 2018.[3]

MBS continues to be more effective than conventional management for weight loss in patients suffering from clinically severe obesity.[4] This class of procedures is the most effective way to achieve significant, durable weight loss and can lead to amelioration or resolution of most obesity-related comorbidities in adults and adolescents.[5-8] In adolescents affected by clinically severe obesity, MBS may lead to improvements in health and psychosocial well-being that exceed those that would be expected if the operation was delayed until later in life.[9,10]

Overweight and Obesity

Obesity is defined using body mass index (BMI) criteria, calculated as weight (kg)/height $(m)^2$, as shown in Box 1.1.[11,12] This criteria includes the latest guideline suggesting lowering BMI criterion for those of Asian ethnicity due to the risk correlation of type 2 diabetes; however, US insurance companies are not lowering their criterion at this time for this population.[13] The BMI criteria for obesity are subdivided into classes I through III, with class I regarded as low-risk obesity, class II deemed moderate-risk obesity, and class III associated with the highest obesity-related health risks. Class III is often referred to as clinically severe obesity. The prevalence of individuals affected by clinically severe obesity has been increasing at faster rates than in lower BMI classes since 1990.[14]

The utility of using BMI is often debated, and it is critical for clinicians to have a general understanding of the most commonly used techniques for the assessment of adiposity (eg, waist circumference, waist-to-hip ratio, body composition analysis, skinfold thickness, underwater weighing, and dual-energy x-ray absorptiometry).[15] Health care providers should also be able to understand how to interpret these measurements, and there are limitations for each type of analysis, especially when applied to varied populations. Various analysis techniques will provide differing insight into not only percentage body fat but also fat distribution, muscle mass, and bone mass.[16]

Criteria for Metabolic and Bariatric Surgery

In 1991, the National Institutes of Health (NIH) Consensus Development Conference Panel developed the criteria for MBS.[17] Although new

BOX 1.1 Classification of Body Weight According to Body Mass Index[11-13]

Adults body mass index (BMI)

	All ethnicities except Asian	Asian ethnicity
Underweight	less than 18.5	less than 18.5
Normal or acceptable weight	18.5 to 24.9	18.5 to 22.9
Overweight	25 to 29.9	23 to 24.9
Obesity	30 or greater	25 or greater
Obesity Class I	30 to 34.9	25 to 29.9
Obesity Class II		30 or greater
Obesity Class III (clinically severe obesity)	40 or higher	—

Children (aged 2 to 18 years) BMI-for-age percentile growth chart

Underweight	less than 5th percentile
Normal or healthy weight	5th percentile to 85th percentile
Overweight	85th percentile to 95th percentile
Obesity	95th percentile or greater

surgical techniques and procedures have been developed since then, the current criteria for MBS deviate little from these recommendations. Box 1.2 on page 4 lists the criteria originally recommended by the NIH and some additional requirements by many insurers.[17,18] See Chapter 6 for criteria and preoperative and postoperative care of adolescent MBS patients.

BOX 1.2 Qualifications for Consideration of Metabolic and Bariatric Surgery[13,17-23]

Inclusion criteria

Body mass index (BMI) 40 or greater, or more than 100 lb overweight.

BMI 35 or greater with comorbid conditions[a] (at least one, such as type 2 diabetes, hypertension, sleep apnea and other respiratory disorders, nonalcoholic fatty liver disease, osteoarthritis, lipid abnormalities, gastrointestinal disorders, or heart disease).

Of note, laparoscopic adjustable gastric band (AGB) is a US Food and Drug Administration–approved option for those patients with a BMI 30 or greater with one comorbid condition.

Inability to achieve and sustain a healthy weight loss for a period of time with prior weight loss efforts.

Also recommended

The National Institutes of Health as well as the American College of Surgeons and the American Society for Metabolic and Bariatric Surgery also recommend that surgery be performed:

- by a board-certified surgeon with specialized training or experience in bariatric and metabolic surgery or
- at a center that has a multidisciplinary team of experts for follow-up care (this may include a nutritionist, exercise physiologist or specialist, and a mental health professional).

Some insurance companies require that the surgery be performed at a facility that is accredited by the Metabolic and Bariatric Surgery Accreditation and Quality Improvement Program (MBSAQIP).

[a] Clinical Practice Guidelines (2019) state that patients with a BMI of 30 to 34.9 and type 2 diabetes mellitus with inadequate glycemic control despite optimizing lifestyle and medical therapy should be considered for a bariatric procedure. Current evidence is insufficient to support recommending a metabolic and bariatric procedure in the absence of obesity. See reference 13.

Types of Bariatric Surgery

Metabolic and bariatric procedures are grouped according to their mechanisms of action and were previously referred to as either restrictive or malabsorptive procedures, with some procedures characterized by both mechanisms of action.[17,24] However, to truly understand the mechanisms of MBS, these complex metabolic changes should be considered[25]:

- **Nonmetabolic operations provide significant weight loss without altering the physiology of energy (fat) storage.** One example includes the adjustable gastric band (AGB) procedure (see Figure 1.1 on page 6).
- **Metabolic procedures that include gastric manipulation have a profound effect on the secretion of gut hormones that lead to decreased hunger and increased satiety.** These procedures include the Roux-en-Y gastric bypass (RYGB) (see Figure 1.2 on page 7) and the sleeve gastrectomy (SG) (see Figure 1.3 on page 8). Research on the impact of metabolic and gastric manipulation procedures on changes to gut-brain communication is ongoing. Changes in gastric manipulation may decrease hydrochloric acid production in the stomach, which may hinder nutrient absorption.[26-28]
- **Metabolic procedures cause severe malabsorption of nutrients.** These procedures result in significant intestinal malabsorption of protein, calories, and micronutrients, as well as changes in the secretion of gut hormones that lead to decreased hunger and increased satiety. These surgical procedures include the biliopancreatic diversion (BPD) (not illustrated) and the BPD with duodenal switch (BPD/DS) (see Figure 1.4 on page 9). A newer subcategory within the metabolic procedures category includes one anastomosis procedures. The American Society for Metabolic and Bariatric Surgery (ASMBS) recently endorsed the single-anastomosis duodeno-ileostomy with sleeve (SADI-S) (see Figure 1.5 on page 10), and this procedure will likely be aligned closer to the RYGB than the BPD/DS regarding micronutrient malabsorption, but more research is necessary.[29] The one-anastomosis gastric bypass (OAGB) (see Figure 1.6 on page 11) is not endorsed by the

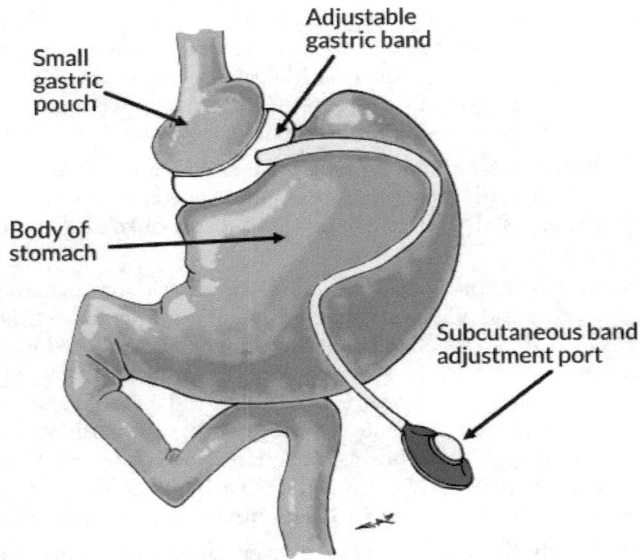

FIGURE 1.1 Adjustable gastric band (AGB) procedure

An adjustable band is placed around the top of the stomach, reducing the capacity of the stomach, thereby reducing food intake. The band is tethered to tubing attached to a port that is placed just under the skin. The port provides access for saline to be injected in small amounts over time to allow for adequate restriction of food intake by filling the balloon inside the band. Adjustments are completed as necessary to adjust the volume of food intake, ensure food tolerance, and help patients feel full sooner and stay full longer.
Illustrations reprinted with permission by Dr. Edo Aarts, MD, PhD.

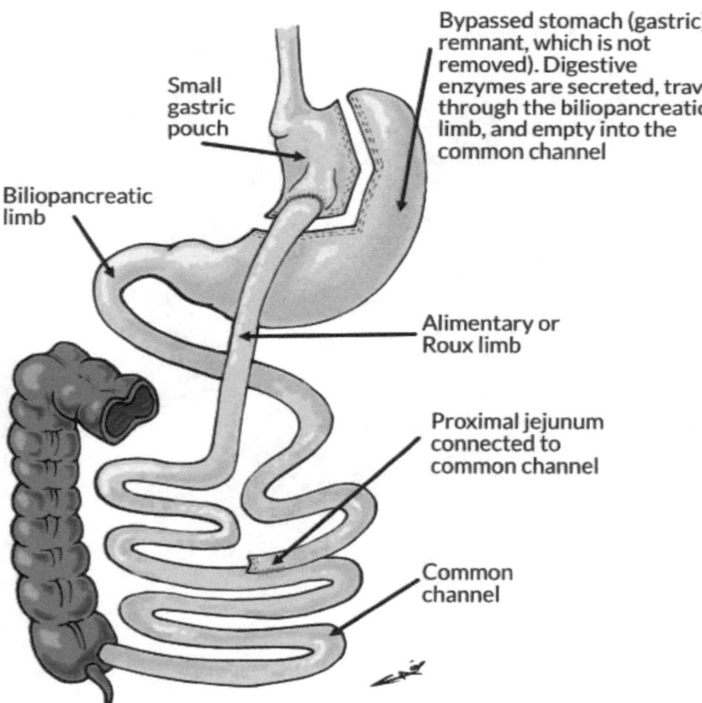

FIGURE 1.2 Roux-en-Y gastric bypass (RYGB) procedure

In the laparoscopic procedure, the stomach is divided into two parts, thereby creating a small pouch (the proximal pouch of the stomach) and a larger excluded pouch (remnant portion of the stomach). Part of the small intestine is bypassed creating the intestinal "short" Roux limb. The bypassed intestine is attached to the proximal pouch.
Illustrations reprinted with permission by Dr. Edo Aarts, MD, PhD.

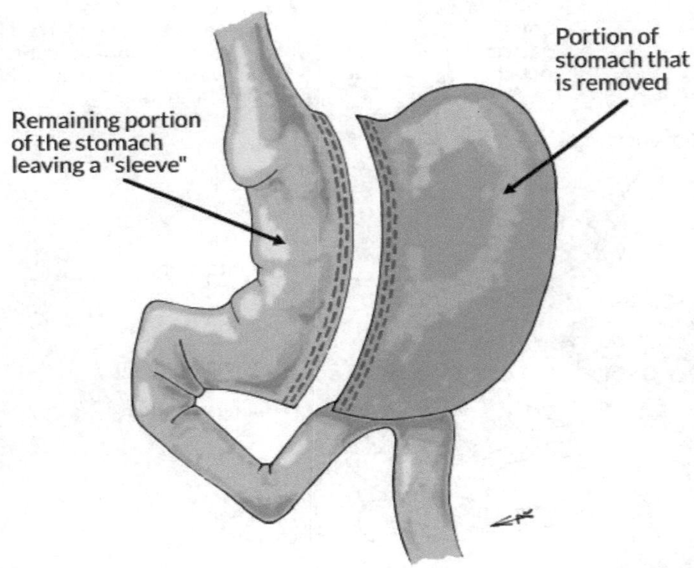

FIGURE 1.3 Sleeve gastrectomy (SG) procedure

In this procedure, about 75% to 80% of the stomach (the fundus) is removed, leaving what resembles a "sleeve" or a narrow tube. The pyloric sphincter and intestines remain intact, so the food pathway is not altered.

Illustrations reprinted with permission by Dr. Edo Aarts, MD, PhD.

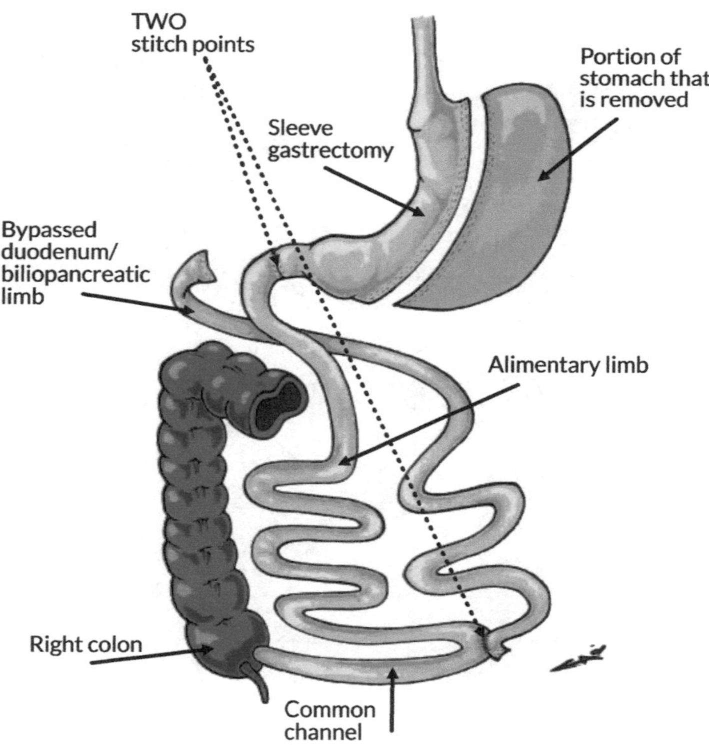

FIGURE 1.4 Biliopancreatic diversion with duodenal switch (BPD/DS) procedure

Roughly 75% to 80% of the stomach is permanently removed, similar to a sleeve gastrectomy. The pylorus, which is the valve at the outlet of the stomach, remains intact. The stomach is then connected to the last 250 cm (~8 feet) of small intestine. The remainder of the small intestine is connected 75 to 150 cm from the end of the small bowel, forming the common channel, where food mixes with the digestive enzymes.
Illustrations reprinted with permission by Dr. Edo Aarts, MD, PhD.

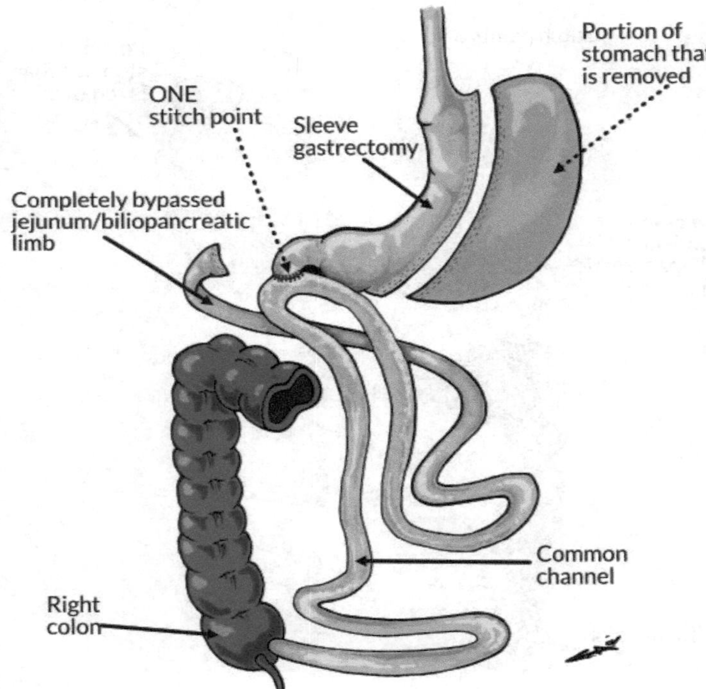

FIGURE 1.5 Single-anastomosis duodeno-ileostomy with sleeve (SADI-S) procedure

Roughly 75% to 80% of the stomach is permanently removed, similar to a sleeve gastrectomy.. The pylorus, which is the valve at the outlet of the stomach, remains intact. Unlike the biliopancreatic diversion with duodenal switch, the SADI-S completely bypasses the jejenum and leaves very little duodenum and some of the ileum. The remainder of the small intestine is connected 250 to 300 cm from the end of the small bowel, forming the common channel, where food mixes with the digestive enzymes.
Illustrations reprinted with permission by Dr. Edo Aarts, MD, PhD.

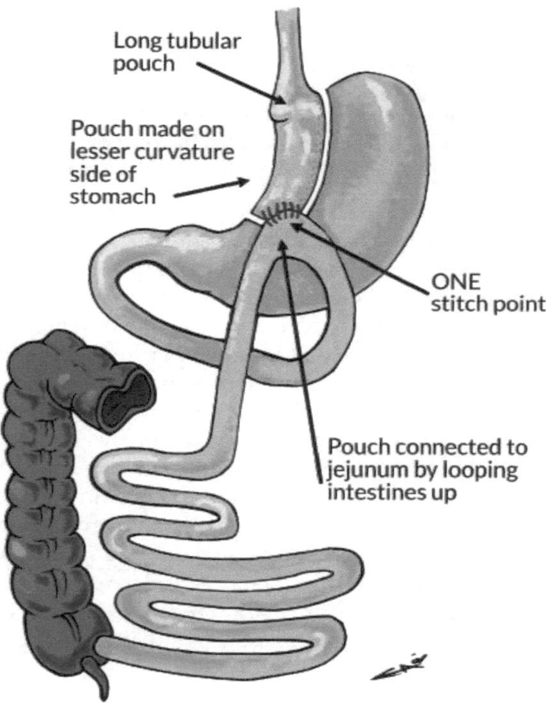

FIGURE 1.6 One-anastomosis gastric bypass (OAGB) procedure

A long tubular pouch is made on the lesser curvature of the stomach. The pouch is then connected to a loop of the jejunum portion of the small intestine at roughly 150 to 250 cm from the ligament of Treitz.

Illustrations reprinted with permission by Dr. Edo Aarts, MD, PhD.

by the ASMBS; however, it is growing in popularity worldwide with a very small number being performed in the United States. In addition, patients are traveling to other countries to get this procedure, more commonly referred to as mini-gastric bypass (MGB); however, the OAGB is a modification of the original version of an MGB. Therefore, a brief overview of these procedures should be provided if care is needed for these patients.

Procedure variation of recommendations for necessary vitamin and mineral supplementation is expected due to the metabolic changes and gastric manipulation by surgery type. Some patients may require additional supplementation due to their procedure having an increased need for certain nutrients due to higher rates of malabsorption or the inability to absorb certain nutrients as compared with other procedures. Food intolerance may also play a role when it comes to individual patient variation regarding necessary supplementation. Most importantly, it is critical to evaluate each patient by reviewing their medical history, medication usage (to evaluate for potential drug-nutrient interactions), food intake, MBS history, biochemical analysis, and any signs or symptoms of potential deficiencies. See Appendix C for information regarding vitamin and mineral requirements. Appendix D includes recommended biochemical surveillance to assist with evaluating and treating potential nutrient deficiencies. For further information regarding tips on educating and counseling patients that may assist with enhancing supplement adherence, see Appendix H.

Each procedure has variable, but often profound, effects on weight and comorbidity. Investigation of the changes that occur due to the manipulation of the stomach or digestive tract due to MBS has been ongoing over the past couple of decades. The mechanisms of action and metabolic changes associated with the various types of MBS are not completely understood. Recent data suggest that the RYGB, in addition to affecting neural and hormonal pathways, also affects gut microbiota.[30] Box 1.3 describes the characteristics of the gut hormones that have been the most studied.[24,31-37]

BOX 1.3 Gut Hormones and Their Role in Metabolic and Bariatric Surgery[24,31-38]

Glucagon-like peptide-1

Mechanism

Acts synergistically with peptide YY: induces satiety and inhibits food intake

Augments the insulin response to nutrients

Slows gastric emptying

Inhibits glucagon secretion

Postoperative effect

Sleeve gastrectomy (SG), Roux-en-Y gastric bypass (RYGB), biliopancreatic diversion with duodenal switch (BPD/DS), and single-anastomosis duodeno-ileostomy with sleeve (SADI-S): increased

Adjustable gastric band (AGB): no effect or increased (conflicting data)

Peptide YY

Mechanism

Inhibitory effect on gastrointestinal motility

Shown to induce satiety and reduce food intake

Postoperative effect

SG, RYGB, and BPD/DS: increased

AGB: no effect

SADI-S: unknown

Ghrelin

Mechanism

Produced from the fundus of the stomach and the proximal intestine

Only known orexigenic ("hunger") hormone in the gut

Primary source is the gastric mucosa

Nutrient exposure to the small intestine is sufficient for food-induced ghrelin suppression in human beings; therefore, gastric nutrient exposure is not necessary for suppression.

Continued on next page

BOX 1.3 Gut Hormones and Their Role in Metabolic and Bariatric Surgery[24,31-38] (cont.)

Postoperative effect

AGB: increased

RYGB: decreased

SG and BPD/DS: inconclusive

SADI-S: unknown

Weight Loss Outcomes of Surgery

Since obesity is a complicated condition of weight regulation and the causes of obesity vary, obesity therapy outcomes, including surgery outcomes, also vary. In addition, weight loss outcomes are reported in multiple ways, including:

- excess weight loss (EWL) (eg, in pounds or kilograms),
- the percentage of excess weight loss (%EWL),
- total body weight loss (TBWL), and
- the percentage of total body weight loss (%TBWL).

Registered dietitian nutritionists (RDNs) must be aware of how %EWL is calculated and be able to distinguish among these four terms in the literature. Box 1.4 explains how to determine a patient's excess body weight (EBW) prior to MBS, the %EWL after surgery, TBWL, and %TBWL. Table 1.1 on page 17 shows weight loss by procedure as %EWL and %TBWL at 2, 10, and 20 years postoperatively.[5,7,39]

Morbidity and Mortality Outcomes of Surgery

Surgical operations for weight loss are often considered both metabolic and bariatric (or bariatric in the case of the AGB) surgeries because, as

BOX 1.4 Calculating Excess Body Weight Before Bariatric Surgery and Percentage of Excess Weight Loss and Total Body Weight Loss

Excess body weight (EBW)

To determine a patient's EBW prior to metabolic and bariatric surgery:

1. Calculate what a patient's weight would be if body mass index (BMI) were 25.

$$25 \times \frac{\text{height in inches}^2}{703} = \text{weight in lb to be at BMI of 25}$$

   Online BMI calculators may be helpful in this determination

2. Subtract that weight from the patient's actual weight before metabolic and bariatric surgery.

   Example: Patient's preoperative weight is 320 lb and their height is 5′7″ (67″)

$$\text{BMI of } 25 = 25 \times \frac{67^2}{703} = 159.6 \text{ lb}$$

$$\text{EBW} = 320 \text{ lb} - 159.6 \text{ lb} = 160.4 \text{ lb}$$

Percentage of excess weight loss (%EWL)

To determine %EWL after metabolic and bariatric surgery:

1. Measure the amount of weight lost after surgery.
2. Divide that amount by the amount of preoperative excess body weight.
3. Multiply by 100.

   Example using the previously referenced patient that now weighs 200 lb postoperatively:

$$320 \text{ lb} - 200 \text{ lb} = 120 \text{ lb}$$

$$\frac{120 \text{ lb}}{160.4 \text{ lb}} \times 100 = 74.8\% \text{ EWL}$$

Continued on next page

BOX 1.4 Calculating Excess Body Weight Before Bariatric Surgery and Percentage of Excess Weight Loss and Total Body Weight Loss (cont.)

Percentage of total body weight loss (%TBWL)

To determine a patient's %TBWL after metabolic and bariatric surgery:

1. Subtract the patient's current weight from their preoperative weight.
2. Divide that by their preoperative weight.
3. Multiply by 100.

   Example using the same patient mentioned earlier (320 lb preoperatively; currently 200 lb):

$$\frac{320\text{ lb} - 200\text{ lb}}{320\text{ lb}} \times 100 = 37.5\%\text{TBWL}$$

noted, they not only lead to significant weight loss but also influence metabolic processes and, in turn, morbidity and mortality outcomes. There is now a large body of scientific evidence demonstrating remission of type 2 diabetes mellitus (T2DM) following MBS. A large review of 621 studies that included more than 135,247 patients found that MBS results in improvement of T2DM in more than 85% of patients with diabetes and remission of the disease in 78% of patients. Remission was highest for BPD/DS patients at 95%, followed by RYGB patients with remission in 80%, and AGB patients reporting a remission rate of 60%. Other studies found comparable rates between SG and RYGB (ie, 80% remission).[43] SADI-S has been reported to have a resolution rate of 74.1% for T2DM.[44] Other morbidity outcomes for the four most common procedures combined (AGB, SG, RYGB, and BPD/DS) plus SADI-S are described in Table 1.2 (see page 18).[44-46]

The differences between procedures were marginal regarding improvement or resolution of comorbid conditions.[46] The mortality rate for MBS is less than 0.3% (3 out of 1,000) and is similar to that of gallbladder removal and considerably less than that of a hip replacement.[43] In fact, Medicare has approved metabolic and bariatric surgical procedures

TABLE 1.1 Weight Loss Outcomes of Metabolic and Bariatric Procedures[5,7,39-42]

Procedure	Weight loss outcomes over time					
	2 years postoperative		10 years postoperative		20 years postoperative	
	%EWL[a]	%TBWL[b]	%EWL	%TBWL	%EWL	%TBWL
AGB[c]	52.6%	20.4%	45.9%	19.4%	48.9%	22.2%
SG[d]	58%	25%	58.3%	26.3%	ND[e]	
RYGB[f]	68%	35%	56.7%	25%	ND	
BPD/DS[g]	65.1%	ND	74.1%	ND	ND	
	1 year postoperative		2 years postoperative		5 years postoperative	
	%EWL	%TBWL	%EWL	%TBWL	%EWL	%TBWL
SADI-S[f]	72%	38.6%	ND	38.7%	ND	37%

[a] % EWL = percentage of excess weight loss
[b] % TBWL = percentage of total body weight loss
[c] AGB = adjustable gastric band
[d] SG = sleeve gastrectomy
[e] ND = no data
[f] RYGB = Roux-en-Y gastric bypass
[g] BPD/DS = biliopancreatic diversion with duodenal switch
[h] SADI-S = single-anastomosis duodeno-ileostomy with sleeve

TABLE 1.2 Morbidity Outcomes 1 Year After Metabolic Bariatric Surgery[44-46]

	Patients achieving improvement/resolution	
Comorbidity	**Four main procedures combined (AGB,[a] SG,[b] RYGB,[c] and BPD/DS[d])**	**SADI-S[e]**
Hypertension	53.2%-68%	96.3%
Dyslipidemia	69.8%-71%	68.3%
Obstructive sleep apnea	66.6%	63.3%
Gastroesophageal reflux	74.4%	87.5%

[a] AGB = adjustable gastric band
[b] SG = sleeve gastrectomy
[c] RYGB = Roux-en-Y gastric bypass
[d] BPD/DS = biliopancreatic diversion with duodenal switch
[e] SADI-S = single-anastomosis duodeno-ileostomy with sleeve

based on data that showed a 7-year increase in life expectancy for individuals undergoing metabolic and bariatric surgery.[47]

There are more than 15 randomized controlled trials (RCTs), which are the highest standards for research protocols, discussing comorbidity outcomes of T2DM remission after bariatric surgery. Reports of T2DM remission among postoperative MBS patients have varied. Table 1.3 summarizes five RCTs showing diabetes remission following MBS.[48]

Procedure Choice

In the United States, experts estimate that more than 250,000 patients had surgery in 2018; SG was ranked as the most performed procedure. SG has been the most popular MBS option for more than 5 years.[3] RYGB and revision are nearly tied for second place at somewhere between 15% and 20%, with all other procedures ranging from less than 1% to 2%.[3] The most common procedures will be focused on more closely in this pocket guide, with brief overviews of the other procedures.

TABLE 1.3 Summary of Randomized Controlled Trials Showing Diabetes Remission Following Metabolic and Bariatric Surgery[20,48-53]

Author/ year	Country	Sample size (n)	Follow-up (months)	Surgery type	Type 2 diabetes mellitus remission rate	
					Bariatric	Conventional
O'Brien et al, 2006[49]	Australia	80	24	Adjustable gastric band	93%	46.7%
Dixon et al, 2008[20]	Australia	60	24	Adjustable gastric band	73%	13%
Mingrone et al, 2012[50]	Italy	60	24	Roux-en-Y gastric bypass & biliopancreatic diversion with duodenal switch	85%	0%
Schauer et al, 2012[51]	United States	150	12	Roux-en-Y gastric bypass & sleeve gastrectomy	39.4%	12%
Schauer et al, 2017[52]	United States	[a]	[a]	Roux-en-Y gastric bypass & sleeve gastrectomy	50%[a]	21%
Ikramuddin et al, 2013[53]	United States	120	12	Roux-en-Y gastric bypass	49%	19%

[a] Please review article for more clear data points as Roux-en-Y gastric bypass and sleeve gastrectomy were evaluated separately in this study but combined for clearer presentation purposes.

The MBS options offered to today's patient vary in their rate of postoperative weight loss, remission, or improvement of obesity-related comorbid conditions, nutritional requirements, and nature and severity of complications. There is no perfect procedure, and it is critical that an informed risk and benefit assessment should be made by each patient.[54] The choice of having MBS and then choosing which procedure ultimately depends on factors related to individual risk/benefit analysis. For further information regarding determining the risk/benefit analysis, visit the American College of Surgeons website to utilize their bariatric surgical risk/benefit calculator.[55]

The Role of the Registered Dietitian Nutritionist

The RDN is responsible for the nutrition care of the MBS patient and plays an important role in every aspect of care, from preoperative assessment and education of the patient to long-term follow-up, evaluation, and monitoring. There are few standardized recommendations for postoperative RDN visits, and nutrition protocols vary greatly among surgical centers. Therefore, RDNs working in a metabolic and bariatric practice should set up standard postoperative nutrition protocols appropriate for that practice (see Figure 1.7 for suggestions; only the four most common procedures were included in this data set).[13]

All patients should have access to a bariatric-trained RDN. The visits described later are merely for suggestion to assist with standardizing medical nutrition therapy (MNT) visits across surgical centers. Long-term RDN-provided MNT is helpful to assist with returning hunger, weight regain, and mitigating the risk of nutritional deficiencies.[56,57] Patients may benefit from any combination of one-on-one visits with the RDN, group visits (or classes), or support groups provided by the surgical center. All three types of visits may be in-person or may be provided through telemedicine to increase patient efficacy and potentially enhance patient outcomes.

	AGB	SG	RYGB	BPD/DS
Early Postoperative Care				
1. Protocol-derived staged meal progression	X	X	X	X
2. Healthy eating education	X	X	X	X
3. Education regarding proper supplementation and nutrient deficiency prevention program	X	X	X	X
4. Hydration education	X	X	X	X
Follow-Up Care				
1. First Visit Postoperatively (X Month Postoperatively)	1	1	1	1
2. Visit Intervals Until Stable (Every X Months)	1-2	3	3	3
3. Visits Once Stable (Months)	12	6, 12	6-12	6
4. Monitor adherence with physical activity recommendations in collaboration with the multi-disciplinary team	X	X	X	X
5. In collaboration with the multidisciplinary team, encourage support group attendance; educate patient on available offerings if needed	X	X	X	X
6. Provide ongoing nutrition education	X	X	X	X
7. Provide ongoing education regarding proper micro-nutrient supplementation and nutrient deficiency prevention	X	X	X	X

FIGURE 1.7 Suggested postoperative care and follow-up of the metabolic and bariatric surgery patient by the registered dietitian nutritionist

Abbreviations: AGB, adjustable gastric band; SG, sleeve gastrectomy; RYGB, Roux-en-Y gastric bypass; BPD/DS, biliopancreatic diversion with duodenal switch; RDN, registered dietitian nutritionist.

Multidisciplinary team may include RDNs, bariatric surgeons, primary care physician, bariatricians, nurse practitioners, physician assistants, behavioral health experts, exercise physiology experts, registered nurses, medical assistants, and so on. See Appendix E for more information.

Adapted from Mechanick JI, Apovian C, Brethauer S, et al. Clinical practice guidelines for the perioperative nutrition, metabolic, and nonsurgical support of patients undergaoin bariatric procedures—2019 update: cosponsored by American Association of Clinical Endocrinologists/American College of Endocrinology, the Obesity Society, American Society for Metabolic & Bariatric Surgery, Obesity Medicine Association, and American Society of Anesthesiologists. *Surg Obes Relat Dis.* 2020;16(2):175-247. doi:10.1016/j.soard.2019.10.02. See reference 13.

Support Groups

Support groups are a critical tool in the care of MBS patients, as they have been shown to improve patient outcomes.[58-61] Support groups can be held for preoperative patients, postoperative patients, or combined for preoperative and postoperative patients. Different modalities can be utilized, such as in-person, virtual, phone conference, or peer-run support groups. The ASMBS Integrated Health Support Group Manual[62] is a valuable resource for support group implementation. No matter the approach, support groups provide an opportunity for RDNs to provide patients with information and deal with unexpected challenges.

Patient-Centered Care

It is the intent of the bariatric RDN to provide patient-centered care to MBS patients. The patient and the RDN work in partnership to meet the patient's health goals.[63] It is the right of every patient to receive respectful, responsive care, and the RDN must take into account individual patient preferences, needs, and values when guiding clinical decisions. Thus, it is of utmost importance for the RDN to utilize the evidence-based practice in this text within the context of the individual patients they are serving. In addition, the RDN is guided by the Academy of Nutrition and Dietetics Code of Ethics for the Nutrition and Dietetics Profession. This includes adherence to "the core values of customer focus, integrity, innovation, social responsibility, and diversity," as well as using "science-based decisions."[64]

Patient-Centered Language

In addition to patient-centered care and following the direction of the Academy of Nutrition and Dietetics Code of Ethics, it is critical that patient-centered language is used when working with patients with obesity and other diseases. Similar references to other individuals avoid defining the patient by their ability or their disease (eg, "disabled person" and "diabetic patient"). The proper terms, "individual with a disability" and "patient with diabetes," should be used; this is commonly referred to as person-first, patient-first, or person-centered language. The RDN and other health care professionals should use person-first language and words that respect and acknowledge an individual as a whole person and avoid the use of describing a patient by their disease. For example, avoid using the term, "obese person," and replace it with "person with obesity." Putting the patient first and the disease second helps eliminate stereotypes.

It is important to note that some clinicians perceive the word "obesity" to have a negative connotation. However, obesity is a medical term, disease diagnosis, and nutrition diagnosis. Therefore, it is a medically appropriate word; however, it is important to be respectful of the preferred language of a patient when communicating with them. Research suggests that individuals with obesity prefer their medical providers to use the words, "BMI" and "weight" when referring to excess adiposity.[65-68]

Weight Bias and Sensitivity Training

In addition to patient-centered language, addressing the issue of weight bias among health care professionals is a critical undertaking. In a sample of 2,449 people with obesity, 69% reported experiencing weight stigma from doctors, 46% from nurses, 37% from RDNs, and 21% from mental health professionals.[69] As such, it is a requirement for a Metabolic and Bariatric Surgery Accreditation and Quality Improvement Program (MBSAQIP) to provide bariatric or obesity sensitivity training to everyone at their institution.[70] These trainings should address the necessity for patient-centered care, person-first language, and identification and awareness of explicit and implicit weight bias among health care professionals working with MBS patients. In order to assess implicit weight bias, visit the Project Implicit website (www.implicit.harvard.edu).[71] Awareness of one's bias is the first step in changing it. Thus, RDNs are uniquely poised to champion for antiweight bias, sensitivity training, and the use of patient-first language in the field of MBS.

References

1. Hales CM, Carroll MD, Fryar CD, Ogden CL. Prevalence of obesity and severe obesity among adults: United States, 2017-2018. NCHS Data Brief, no 360. National Center for Health Statistics. 2020. Accessed March 3, 2020. www.cdc.gov/nchs/products/databriefs/db360.htm
2. Hales CM, Carroll MD, Fryar CD, Ogden CL. Prevalence of obesity among adults and youth: United States, 2015-2016. NCHS Data Brief, no 288. National Center for Health Statistics. 2017. Accessed March 3, 2020. www.cdc.gov/nchs/data/databriefs/db288.pdf
3. American Society of Metabolic and Bariatric Surgery. Estimate of bariatric surgery numbers, 2011-2018. ASMBS. June 2018. Accessed March 3, 2020. https://asmbs.org/resources/estimate-of-bariatric-surgery-numbers
4. Colquitt J, Clegg A, Sidhu M, et al. Surgery for morbid obesity. *Cochrane Database Syst Rev.* 2005;4:CD006341. doi:10.1002/14651858.CD003641.pub2
5. Sjostrom L, Lindroos AK, Peltonen M, et al. Lifestyle, diabetes and cardiovascular risk factors 10 years after bariatric surgery. *N Engl J Med.* 2004;351(26):2683-2693. doi:10.1056/NEJMoa035622
6. Hutter MM, Schirmer BD, Jones DB, et al. First report from the American College of Surgeons Bariatric Surgery Center Network: laparoscopic sleeve gastrectomy has morbidity and effectiveness positioned between the band and the bypass. *Ann Surg.* 2011;254(3):410-422. doi:10.1097/SLA.0b013e31822c9dac
7. Buchwald H, Avidor Y, Braunwald E, et al. Bariatric surgery a systematic review and meta-analysis. *JAMA.* 2004;292(14):1724-1737. doi:10.1001/jama.292.14.1724
8. Inge TH, Xanthakos SA, Zeller MH. Bariatric surgery for pediatric extreme obesity: now or later? *Int J Obesity.* 2007;31(1):1-14. doi:10.1038/sj.ijo.0803525
9. Barlow SE; Expert Committee. Expert Committee recommendations regarding the prevention, assessment, and treatment of child and adolescent overweight and obesity: summary report. *Pediatrics.* 2007;120(suppl 4):S164-S192. doi:10.1542/peds.2007-2329C
10. Garcia VF, DeMaria EJ. Adolescent bariatric surgery: treatment delayed, treatment denied, a crisis invited. *Obes Surg.* 2006;16(1):1-4. doi:10.1381/096089206775222195
11. Centers for Disease Control and Prevention. Overweight & obesity: defining adult obesity. CDC. April 2017. Accessed March 3, 2020. www.cdc.gov/obesity/adult/defining.html

12. Centers for Disease Control and Prevention. Healthy weight: about child & teen BMI. CDC. July 2018. Accessed March 3, 2020. www.cdc.gov/healthyweight/assessing/bmi/childrens_bmi/about_childrens_bmi.html
13. Mechanick JI, Apovian C, Brethauer S, et al. Clinical practice guidelines for the perioperative nutrition, metabolic, and nonsurgical support of patients undergaoin bariatric procedures—2019 update: cosponsored by American Association of Clinical Endocrinologists/American College of Endocrinology, the Obesity Society, American Society for Metabolic & Bariatric Surgery, Obesity Medicine Association, and American Society of Anesthesiologists. *Surg Obes Relat Dis.* 2020;16(2):175-247. doi:10.1016/j.soard.2019.10.025
14. Finkelstein EA, Khavjou OA, Thompson H, et al. Obesity and severe obesity forecasts through 2030. *Am J Prev Med.* 2012;42(6):563-570. doi:10.1016/j.amepre.2011.10.026
15. American Association of Nurse Practitioners. Modalities to evaluate adiposity. AANP. 2018. Accessed December 30, 2020. https://aapa.org/wp-content/uploads/2018/09/Modalities-to-Evaluate-Adiposity.pdf
16. Cornier MA, Despres JP, Davis N, et al. Assessing Adiposity. *Circulation.* 2011;124(18):1996-2019. doi:10.1161/CIR.0b013e318233bc6a
17. Grundy SM, Barondess JA, Bellegie NJ, et al.; National Institutes of Health. Gastrointestinal surgery for severe obesity consensus statement. NIH. March 1991. Accessed March 3, 2020. https://consensus.nih.gov/1991/1991GISurgeryObesity084PDF.pdf
18. Karmali S, Stoklossa CJ, Sharma A, et al. Bariatric Surgery: a primer. *Can Fam Physician.* 2010;56(9):873-879.
19. American Society of Metabolic and Bariatric Surgery. Who is a candidate for bariatric surgery? ASMBS. 2020. Accessed June 21, 2020. https://asmbs.org/patients/who-is-a-candidate-for-bariatric-surgery
20. Dixon JB, O'Brien PE, Playfair J, et al. Adjustable gastric banding and conventional therapy for type 2 diabetes: a randomized controlled trial. *JAMA.* 2008;299:316-323. doi:10.1001/jama.299.3.316
21. Parikh M, Duncombe J, Fielding GA. Laparoscopic adjustable gastric banding for patients with body mass index of < or = 35 kg/m^2. *Surg Obes Relat Dis.* 2006;2:518-522. doi:10.1016/j.soard.2006.07.005
22. Choi J, Digiorgi M, Milone L, et al. Outcomes of laparoscopic adjustable gastric banding in patients with low body mass index. *Surg Obes Relat Dis.* 2010;6:367-371. doi:10.1016/j.soard.2009.09.021
23. FDA: U.S. Food & Drug Administration. FDA approved obesity treatment devices. FDA. 2016. Accessed July 21, 2020. http://wayback.archive-it.org/7993/20170111083348/http://www.fda.gov/MedicalDevices/ProductsandMedicalProcedures/ObesityDevices/ucm350134.htm

24. Mechanick JI, Kushner RF, Sugerman HJ, et al. American Association of Clinical Endocrinologists, the Obesity Society, and American Society for Metabolic and Bariatric Surgery medical guidelines for clinical practice for the perioperative nutritional, metabolic and nonsurgical support of the bariatric surgery patient. *Surg Obes Relat Dis.* 2008;4(5 suppl):S109-S184. doi:10.1016/j.soard.2008.08.009

25. Buchwald H, Fobi MAL, Herron D, et al.; American College of Surgeons; Bulletin. Definition and history of metabolic surgery. ACS. August 2017. Accessed March 3, 2020. https://bulletin.facs.org/2019/01/definition-and-history-of-metabolic-surgery

26. Ben-Porat T, Elazary R, Goldenshluger A, et al. Nutritional deficiencies four years after laparoscopic sleeve gastrectomy—are supplements required for a lifetime? *Surg Obes Relat Dis.* 2017;13(7):1138-1144. doi:10.1016/j.soard.2017.02.021

27. Gehrer S, Kern B, Peters T, et al. Fewer nutrient deficiencies after laparoscopic sleeve gastrectomy (LSG) than after laparoscopic Roux-Y-gastric bypass (LRYGB)-a prospective study. *Obes Surg.* 2010;20(4):447-453. doi:10.1007/s11695-009-0068-4

28. Fujioka K, DiBaise J, Martindale R. Nutrition and metabolic complications after bariatric surgery and their treatment. *J Parenter Enteral Nutr.* 2011;35(5 suppl):52S-59S. doi:10.1177/0148607111413600

29. Kallies K, Rogers AM. American Society for Metabolic and Bariatric Surgery updated statement on single-anastomosis duodenal switch.. *Surg Obes Relat Dis.* Published online March 16, 2020. doi:10.1016/j.soard.2020.03.020

30. Stefater MA, Wilson-Perez HE, Chambers AP, et al. All bariatric surgeries are not created equal: insights from mechanistic comparisons. *Endocr Rev.* 2013;33(4):595-622. doi:10.1210/er.2011-1044

31. Liou AP, Paziuk M, Luevano JM, et al. Conserved shifts in the gut microbiota due to gastric bypass reduce host weight and adiposity. *Sci Transl Med.* 2013;5(178):ra41. doi:10.1126/scitranslmed.3005687

32. Pournaras DJ, le Roux CW. Obesity, gut hormones, and bariatric surgery. *World J Surg.* 2009;33(10):1983-1988. doi:10.1007/s00268-009-0080-9

33. Ochner CN, Gibson C, Shanik N, et al. Changes in neuralhormonal gut peptides following bariatric surgery. *Int J Obes.* 2011;35(2):153-166. doi:10.1038/ijo.2010.132

34. Pereira SS, Guimaraes M, Almeida R, et al. Biliopancreatic diversion with duodenal switch (BPD-DS) and single-anastomosis duodeno-ileal bypass with sleeve gastrectomy (SADI-S) result in distinct post-prandial hormone profiles. *Int J Obes.* 2019;43:2518-2527. doi:10.1038/s41366-018-0282-zRE

35. Baraboi ED, Li W, Labbe SM, et al. Metabolic change induced by the biliopancreatic diversion in diet-induced obesity in male rats: the contributions of sleeve gastrectomy and duodenal switch. *Endocrinology*. 2015;156(4):1316-1329. doi:10.1210/en.2014-1785
36. Dimitriadis GK, Randeva MS, Miras AD. Potential hormone mechanisms of bariatric surgery. *Curr Obes Rep*. 2017;6(3):253-265. doi:10.10007/s13679-017-0276-5
37. Pournaras DJ, le Roux CW. Ghrelin and metabolic surgery. *Int J Pept*. 2010;2010:217267. doi:10.1155/2010/217267
38. Langer FB, Reza Hoda MA, Bohdjalian A, et al. Sleeve gastrectomy and gastric banding: effects on plasma ghrelin levels. *Obes Surg*. 2005;15(7):1024-1029. doi:10.1381/0960892054621125
39. O'Brien PE, Hindle A, Brennan L, et al. Long-term outcomes after bariatric surgery: a systematic review and meta-analysis of weight loss at 10 or more years for all bariatric procedures and a single-centre review of 20-year outcomes after adjustable gastric banding. *Obes Surg*. 2019;29(1):3-14. doi:10.1007/s11695-018-3525-0
40. Felsenreich DM, Langer FB, Kefurt R, et al. Weight loss, weight regain, and conversions to Roux-en-Y Gastric Bypass: 10-year results of laparoscopic sleeve gastrectomy. *Surg Obes Relat Dis*. 2016;12(9):1655-1662. doi:10.1016/j.soard.2016.02.021
41. Sethi M, Chau E, Youn A, et al. Long-term outcomes after biliopancreatic diversion with and without duodenal switch: 2-, 5-, and 10-year data. *Surg Obes Relat Dis*. 2016;12(9):1697-1705. doi:10.1016/j.soard.2016.03.006
42. Topart P, Becouar G. The single anastomosis duodenal switch modifications: a review of the current literature on outcomes. *Surg Obes Relat Dis*. 2017;13(8):1306-1312. doi:10.1016/j.soard.2017.04.027
43. American Society of Metabolic and Bariatric Surgery. Benefits of bariatric surgery. ASMBS. Accessed May 26, 2020. https://asmbs.org/patients/benefits-of-bariatric-surgery
44. Shoar S, Poliakin L, Rubenstein R, et al. Single anastomosis duodeno-ileal switch (SADIS): a systematic review of efficacy and safety. *Obes Surg*. 2018;28(1):104-113. doi:10.1007/s11695-017-2838-8
45. Sudan R, Nguyen NT, Hutter MM, et al. Morbidity, mortality, and weight loss outcomes after reoperative bariatric surgery in the USA. *J Gastrointest Surg*. 2015;19(1):171-178. doi:10.1007/s11605-014-2639-5
46. Heneghan HM, Meron-Eldar S, Brethauer SA, et al. Effect of bariatric surgery on cardiovascular risk profile. *Am J Cardiol*. 2011;108(10):1499-1507. doi:10.1016/j.amjcard.2011.06.076

47. Schauer DP, Arterburn DE, Livingston EH, et al. Impact of bariatric surgery on life expectancy in severely obese patients with diabetes: a decision analysis. *Ann Surg.* 2015;261(5):914-919. doi:10.1097/SLA.0000000000000907
48. Singh AK, Singh R, Kota SK. Bariatric surgery and diabetes remission: who would have thought it? *Indian J Endocrinol Metab.* 2015;19(5):563-576. doi:10.4103/2230-8210.163113
49. O'Brien PE, Dixon JB, Skinner LC, et al. Treatment of mild to moderate obesity with laparoscopic adjustable gastric banding or intensive medical program: a randomized trial. *Ann Intern Med.* 2006;144(9):625-633. doi:10.7326/0003-4819-144-9-200605020-00005
50. Mingrone G, Panunzi S, De Gaetano A, et al. Bariatric surgery versus conventional medical therapy for type 2 diabetes. *N Engl J Med.* 2012;366(17):1577-1585. doi:10.1056/NEJMoa1200111
51. Schauer PR, Kashyap SR, Wolski K, et al. Bariatric surgery versus intensive medical therapy in obese patients with diabetes. *N Engl J Med.* 2012;366(17):1567-1576. doi:10.1056/NEJMoa1200225
52. Schauer PR, Bhatt DL, Kirwan JP, et al. Bariatric surgery versus intensive medical therapy for diabetes—5-year outcomes. *N Engl J Med.* 2017;376(7):641-651. doi:10.1056/NEJMoa1600869
53. Ikramuddin S, Korner J, Lee WJ et al. Roux-en-Y gastric bypass vs intensive medical management for the control of type 2 diabetes, hypertension, and hyperlipidemia: the Diabetes Surgery Study randomized clinical trial. *JAMA.* 2013;309(21):2240-2249. doi:10.1001/jama.2013.5835
54. Kissler HJ, Settmacher U. Bariatric surgery to treat obesity. *Semin Nephrol.* 2013;33(1):75-89. doi:10.1016/j.semnephrol.2012.12.004
55. American College of Surgeons; Metabolic and Bariatric Surgery Accreditation and Quality Improvement Program. Bariatric surgical risk/benefit calculator. ACS. 2020. Accessed July 22, 2020. https://riskcalculator.facs.org/bariatric/patientoutcomes.jsp
56. Endevelt R, Ben-Assuli O, Klain E, et al. The role of the dietitian follow-up in the success of bariatric surgery. *Surg Obes Relat Dis.* 2013;9:963-968. doi:10.1016/j.soard.2013.01.006
57. Sarwer D, Moore R, Spitzer J, et al. A pilot study investigating the efficacy of postoperative dietary counseling to improve outcomes after bariatric surgery. *Surg Obes Relat Dis.* 2012;8:561-568. doi:10.1016/j.soard.2012.02.010
58. Livhits M, Mercado C, Yermilov I, et al. Is social support associated with greater weight loss after bariatric surgery? A systematic review. *Obes Rev.* 2011;12(2):142-148. doi:10.1111/j.1467-789X.2010.00720.x

59. Kaiser KA, Franks SF, Smith AB. Positive relationship between support group attendance and one-year postoperative weight loss in gastric banding patients. *Surg Obes Relat Dis.* 2011;7(1):89-93. doi:10.1016/j.soard.2010.07.013

60. Orth WS, Madan AK, Taddeucci RJ, Coday M, Tichansky DS. Support group meeting attendance is associated with better weight loss. *Obes Surg.* 2008;18(4):391-394. doi:10.1007/s11695-008-9444-8

61. Song Z, Reinhardt K, Buzdon M, Liao P. Association between support group attendance and weight loss after Roux-en-Y gastric bypass. *Surg Obes Relat Dis.* 2008;4(2):100-103. doi:10.1016/j.soard.2007.02.010

62. American Society of Metabolic and Bariatric Surgery. Integrated Health Support Group manual. ASMBS. May 2019. Accessed October 12, 2020. https://asmbs.org/app/uploads/2015/07/ASMBS-Support-Group-Manual-2019.pdf

63. Institute of Medicine (US) Committee on Quality of Health Care in America. *Crossing the Quality Chasm: A New Health System for the 21st Century.* National Academies Press; 2001.

64. Academy of Nutrition and Dietetics. Code of ethics for the nutrition and dietetics profession. June 1, 2018. Accessed October 12, 2020. www.eatrightpro.org/practice/code-of-ethics/what-is-the-code-of-ethics

65. Wadden TA, Didie E. What's in a name? Patients' preferred terms for describing obesity. *Obes Res.* 2003;11(9):1140-1146. doi:10.1038/oby.2003.155

66. Volger S, Vetter ML, Dougherty M, et al. Patients' preferred terms for describing their excess weight: discussing obesity in clinical practice. *Obesity (Silver Spring).* 2012;20(1):147-150. doi:10.1038/oby.2011.217

67. Puhl RM. What words should we use to talk about weight? A systematic review of quantitative and qualitative studies examining preferences for weight-related terminology. *Obes Rev.* 2020;21:e13008. doi:10.1111/obr.13008

68. Ivezaj V, Lydecker JA, Grilo CM. Language matters: patients' preferred terms for discussing obesity and disordered eating with health care providers after bariatric surgery. *Obesity (Silver Spring).* 2020;28:1412-1418. doi:10.1002/oby.22868

69. Puhl RM, Brownell KD. Confronting and coping with weight stigma: an investigation of overweight and obese adults. *Obesity (Silver Spring).* 2006;14(10):1802-1815. doi:10.1038/oby.2006.208

70. American College of Surgeons. Metabolic and Bariatric Surgery Accreditation and Quality Improvement Program (MBSAQIP) optimal resources for metabolic and bariatric surgery. 2019. Accessed October 12, 2020. www.facs.org/quality-programs/mbsaqip/standards

71. Harvard School of Public Health. Project Implicit. 2011. Accessed October 10, 2020. https://implicit.harvard.edu/implicit/takeatest.html

Preoperative

CHAPTER 2

Evaluation and Nutrition Care of Preoperative Patients

Introduction

During the preoperative phase, metabolic and bariatric surgery (MBS) patients undergo surgical, medical, psychological, and nutrition evaluation. In addition to program requirements, patients who are using insurance benefits will need to meet insurance requirements. Some insurance providers will not authorize surgery until patients participate in a medically supervised weight loss program.

The registered dietitian nutritionist (RDN) has a crucial role in preparing the patient for optimal surgical success. At this point, the RDN provides nutrition education and counseling to help patients understand the necessary lifestyle changes, improve weight-related conditions, and resolve vitamin and mineral deficiencies. They also help manage patient expectations for outcomes.

Preoperative Evaluation

The Clinical Practice Guidelines published in 2019 were a collaboration of the American Association of Clinical Endocrinologists (AACE), The

Obesity Society (TOS), American Society for Metabolic and Bariatric Surgery (ASMBS), Obesity Medicine Association (OMA), and American Society of Anesthesiologists (ASA). These practice guidelines recommend that the preoperative work-up includes a comprehensive medical history, psychosocial-behavioral evaluation, clinical nutrition evaluation, and laboratory testing.[1]

Medical Evaluation

The preoperative medical evaluation includes assessment of obesity-related conditions and causes of obesity.[1] The evaluation may be conducted by a bariatric surgeon, an obesity medicine specialist, or an advanced practice provider specializing in obesity management. Box 2.1 provides an overview of the data collected during the initial medical evaluation.

BOX 2.1 Components of Preoperative Medical Evaluation[1]

Complete history and physical reviewing obesity-related conditions, causes of obesity, weight history, and possible contraindications to surgery

Physical examination including measurement of height and weight, calculation of body mass index, evaluation of blood pressure, pulse, and respiration rate

Cardiopulmonary evaluation with sleep apnea screening

Gastrointestinal evaluation

Endocrine evaluation

Pregnancy test

Laboratory tests to evaluate vitamin and mineral status and determine the need for additional testing[a]

[a] See Box 2.5 on page 35 for more information.

Surgical Evaluation

The bariatric surgeon conducts a surgical evaluation (see Box 2.2 on page 32). An important component of the surgical evaluation is the selection of surgery. This decision is made together through consideration

BOX 2.2 Components of Preoperative Surgical Evaluation[1]

Physical examination

Review of past medical and surgical history

Selection of the type of surgery and the surgical procedure based on patient preference and analysis of all presurgical evaluations

of patient preferences and desired health outcomes, expertise of the surgeon and institution, results of the integrated health team's evaluation, and personalized risk stratification.[1] To provide valuable insight for the surgery selection process, the RDN should understand the types of surgery, mechanisms of actions, and outcomes on comorbidities and weight (see Chapter 1).

Following the evaluations from the interdisciplinary team, the final clearance to proceed with surgery is generally provided by the surgeon who will perform the procedure. At this time, medical need has been established, no medical or psychological contraindications have been identified, medical comorbidities are well managed, and the patient has expressed good understanding and commitment to the planned surgical intervention.[1]

Psychosocial Evaluation

The primary goal of a preoperative psychological evaluation is to identify risk factors or potential postoperative challenges that could negatively impact surgical outcomes (see Box 2.3). The evaluation may lead to recommendations of additional management or intervention before or after surgery. It also serves to develop trust and rapport between the clinician and patient for a long-term supportive relationship after surgery. The psychological evaluation may be performed by a licensed behavioral health clinician who specializes in the field of obesity, MBS, or eating disorders.[2] The behavioral health clinician and RDN work closely together for assessment and treatment of disordered eating behaviors and health-related behaviors that could limit a patient from achieving optimal outcomes after surgery.

BOX 2.3 Components of Preoperative Psychosocial Evaluation[2]

Weight history
Current and past history of eating disorders, such as binge eating, night eating syndrome, compensatory behaviors, anorexia nervosa
Psychiatric history and psychosocial functioning
Developmental and family history
Current and past mental health treatment
Cognitive functioning
Personality traits and temperament
Current stressors
Social support
Quality of life
Substance use
Physical activity
Sleep hygiene
Patient motivation and knowledge, including weight loss expectations

Nutrition Evaluation

A preoperative nutrition assessment guides the RDN's nutrition diagnoses and intervention recommendations.[3] This clinical interview allows the RDN to learn about the patient's weight history, current eating behaviors, social support system, and MBS knowledge to gather information to determine the patient's nutritional status and to manage expectations for life after surgery.[3,4] This is also an opportunity to establish rapport with the patient and to promote the value of a lifelong relationship with the bariatric team.

Box 2.4 on page 34 shows data the RDN should collect or analyze during the preoperative nutrition assessment.[3,4] See Figure E.1 on page 270 for a preoperative nutrition evaluation template using the Nutrition Care Process (NCP).

BOX 2.4 Components of Preoperative Nutrition Assessment[3,4]

Anthropometrics: height, weight, body mass index

List of previous weight loss attempts, including the following:

- commercial programs
- medical programs, including weight loss medications and behavior modification group programs
- medical nutrition therapy
- self-directed diets

Weight history, including highest and lowest adult weights

Dietary history (24-hour food intake or food frequency)

Supplement use (including vitamins, minerals, or dietary supplements)

Cultural and social history factors related to weight and diet

Eating behaviors

Meal/snack patterns

Sleep hygiene

Physical activity, including the following:

- sedentary time (hours/day)
- exercise patterns (ie, type of exercise, time spent exercising per day, number of days of activity per week)

Knowledge of metabolic and bariatric surgery (MBS), including weight expectations and impact of surgery on current eating behaviors and habits

Laboratory data about vitamin and mineral status (from the medical evaluation), with focus on micronutrients that can be affected by the specific bariatric procedure as well as potential deficiencies that will need to be repleted before MBS

Biochemical Surveillance

The RDN should assess the findings of the laboratory studies listed in Box 2.5 in the preoperative nutrition evaluation.[1,5]

Food/Nutrition-Related History

The preoperative nutrition evaluation includes a food/nutrition-related history. Items in the history include assessment of nutrient intake, eating patterns, and nutrition management.

BOX 2.5 Preoperative Laboratory Studies[1,5]

Liver function tests
Lipid profile
Complete blood count with differential
Hemoglobin A1c
Serum iron, ferritin, and total iron-binding capacity
Serum vitamin B12 and methylmalonic acid
Serum vitamin B1 (thiamin)
Red blood cell (RBC) folate and serum homocysteine
Intact parathyroid hormone, 25-hydroxyvitamin D, serum alkaline phosphatase
Retinol-binding protein and plasma retinol (vitamin A status)
Plasma a-tocopherol (vitamin E status)
Des-gamma-carboxy prothrombin (vitamin K status)
Serum zinc or RBC zinc[a]
Serum copper or ceruloplasmin[a]

[a] Indicated only in patients having Roux-en-Y gastric bypass or biliopancreatic diversion with duodenal switch.

Preoperative

Nutrient Intake and Eating Patterns

The nutrient intake assessment includes information on overall energy intake, protein-rich foods, calorically dense foods, nutritive quality of foods, and alcohol consumption. The RDN should assess intake patterns, with attention to the following:

- meals eaten away from home
- frequency of eating including all meals and snacks
- pace of eating
- disordered eating patterns, such as binge eating, night eating, and grazing
- emotional, habitual, and other nonhunger triggers for eating

Nutrition Management

The nutrition history also should include aspects of the client's nutrition management, including:

- nutrition knowledge and attitudes;
- weight loss readiness;
- confidence, readiness, and motivation to make behavior changes;
- self-monitoring abilities;
- social and family support; and
- economic and time limitations related to the purchase or preparation of food.

Energy Requirements

Energy requirements can be assessed most accurately using indirect calorimetry. In the absence of indirect calorimetry, resting metabolic rate (RMR) can be estimated using the Mifflin-St. Jeor equation and the client's actual body weight, as shown in Box 2.6.[3]

Box 2.6 Mifflin-St. Jeor Formula for Estimating Resting Metabolic Rate[a,6]

Men resting metabolic rate in kcal/d = (10 × weight in kg) + (6.25 × height in cm) − (5 × age in years) + 5

Women resting metabolic rate in kcal/d = (10 × weight in kg) + (6.25 × height in cm) − (5 × age in years) − 161

[a] Specific recommendations for transgender and gender-diverse people were not provided.

To estimate total energy needs, the RMR is multiplied by a physical activity factor as outlined in the following[3]:

- sedentary: 1.0 to 1.39
- low active: 1.4 to 1.59
- active: 1.6 to 1.89
- very active: 1.9 to 2.5

Nutrition-Related Physical Findings

In addition to reviewing laboratory data, the RDN should identify physical factors that suggest nutrient deficits. Appendix D lists a selection of physical findings that may be noted in the medical evaluation or witnessed by the RDN.

Nutrition Intervention

After completing the nutrition assessment, the RDN determines a nutrition intervention.[3] Common preoperative interventions include weight stabilization or loss; addressing vitamin and mineral deficiencies; improvement of glycemic management; and education on nutrition, lifestyle, and behavioral changes.[1]

Preoperative Diets and Weight Loss

Research does not support a mandate of weight loss for all patients prior to MBS.[7,8] With surgery being the most effective intervention for obesity, withholding it until an arbitrary degree of weight loss is achieved is considered an inappropriate and potentially harmful practice.[8] A surgeon or program may prescribe weight loss in specific cases, such as a patient with a body weight that exceeds the weight limit of the program's equipment or a patient with a body weight distribution that will increase the risks associated with surgery.[1]

The RDN can help patients establish goals that promote weight stabilization before surgery and instill healthy habits that will likely contribute to success after surgery. These goals should be developed collaboratively with the patient and may address nutrient density of the diet, protein-based meals, structured eating patterns, eating behaviors that will prevent gastrointestinal distress, and increased physical activity.[9]

Independent of weight loss, a short-term, low-carbohydrate diet can reduce liver glycogen stores resulting in liver volume reduction and improved access to the stomach during surgery. These diets can be a mix of meal replacements, protein shakes, and real foods. They are effective when prescribed for the 2 weeks leading up to surgery with a daily carbohydrate intake of less than 50 g and individualized daily calorie restriction to prevent weight gain.[10-12]

Repletion of Vitamin and Mineral Deficits

Patients seeking MBS may have vitamin and mineral deficiencies that need to be identified and corrected before surgery.[1,5] See Appendix D for examples of potential micronutrient deficiencies related to obesity as well as repletion guidelines.

Glycemic Management

Blood glucose management before MBS can reduce the risk of postoperative infections and promote wound healing. The AACE/TOS/ASMBS guidelines encourage optimization of blood glucose through medical nutrition therapy, physical activity, and pharmacotherapy and have recommended the glycemic targets listed in Box 2.7.[1] Considering that surgery is a recognized treatment for type 2 diabetes mellitus, individualization of targets is crucial to ensure that patients who can benefit from surgery are not unnecessarily prevented from receiving it.[13]

BOX 2.7 Glycemic Targets Before Metabolic and Bariatric Surgery[1]

Hemoglobin A1c

Desired goal is hemoglobin A1c(HbA1c) 7.0% or less

HbA1c of 7% to 8% should be considered for patients with advanced microvascular or macrovascular complications, extensive comorbid conditions, or long-standing diabetes where intensive efforts have not produced lower HbA1c

For patients with HbA1c more than 8%, clinical judgment needed to proceed with surgery

Blood glucose levels

Fasting blood glucose: 110 mg/dL or less

2-hour postprandial blood glucose: 140 mg/dL or less

Preoperative Carbohydrate Loading

Enhanced recovery after MBS protocols have been implemented in the field of colorectal surgery for several years and are credited with converting inpatient surgeries to day surgeries.[14] These protocols are now being applied in the field of MBS. Enhanced recovery protocols rely on the collaboration of the patient, interdisciplinary team, and institution administration. They include multiple interventions at all phases of surgery. Common interventions include prehabilitation, skin prep prior to surgery, tight glycemic management, scheduled dosing of nonopioid analgesics before and after surgery and minimizing the use of fluids, tubes, and drains intraoperatively as well as postoperative radiologic studies.[15] In a study with 36 participating centers performing Roux-en-Y gastric bypass, sleeve gastrectomy, and adjustable gastric banding surgeries, adherence to an enhanced recovery protocol reduced the length of stay from 2.24 to 1.76 days without an increased risk of bleeding, reoperation, or readmission.[16]

A component of prehabilitation is preoperative carbohydrate loading. Although a minimum of 6 to 8 hours of preoperative fasting is requested by many surgeons and anesthesiologists, technical advances have made this practice questionable. Studies have not demonstrated a greater risk of aspiration with a shortened fast of 2 to 3 hours. Preoperative fasting leads to insulin resistance; a physiological state of stress; and increased thirst, hunger, and anxiety in patients.[17]

Research suggests that oral ingestion of 100 g carbohydrate the night before surgery and 50 g carbohydrate 2 hours before surgery can shift the body from fasting to a fed state. A preferred beverage to achieve this purpose is a clear liquid with 12% carbohydrate coming from complex carbohydrates, such as maltodextrin.[18] There are beverages on the market that have been designed to these exact specifications. However, many MBS programs that are trialing preoperative carbohydrate loading use clear liquid sports drinks or fruit juices.[17] Although it is unclear if this extrapolation of the literature results in the same benefits when compared with a complex carbohydrate beverage, the evidence supporting a shortened preoperative fast is mounting.[14,17]

Nutrition Education and Counseling

Preoperative nutrition education is encouraged to help patients understand the changes they will need to make after surgery. The RDN can provide these nutrition interventions on a one-on-one basis or in small groups. Recommended topics of discussion include :

- the impact of surgery on the gastrointestinal tract,
- eating behaviors to prevent gastrointestinal distress,
- preoperative diet preparation,
- postoperative diet progression, and
- vitamin and mineral supplementation.

Lifestyle and Behavior Changes

Initiation of lifestyle changes can result in weight loss before surgery, which may align with insurance or program requirements. In addition, healthy changes to diet and exercise patterns may position patients for improved long-term postoperative success. Discussing behavior change before surgery allows patients time to become aware of their habits related to food and exercise and make necessary changes for improved postoperative outcomes. Box 2.8 provides examples of preoperative behavior modification and nutrition goals. Appendix H provides information on education and counseling techniques.

Nutrition Care Process Case Study

Box 2.9 on page 42 offers a case study with application of the NCP to the preoperative period.

Health Insurance Requirements

If a patient is using health insurance benefits to subsidize the cost of surgery, they will be required to meet the requirements from the insurance

BOX 2.8 Preoperative Behavior Modification and Nutrition Goals

Behavior modification goals

Follow a structured eating pattern.

Practice mindful eating.

Eat in designated eating areas, preferably without distraction.

Use smaller plates (recommend patients use 7- to 9-inch plates).

Avoid drinking with meals.

Self-monitor eating and physical activity.

Observe environmental cues to nonhunger eating.

Develop awareness of physical hunger and satiety.

Nutrition goals

Decrease/eliminate fast food meals.

Eliminate calorie-containing beverages.

Decrease processed foods and added sugars.

Focus on increasing intake of lean protein foods, whole fruits and vegetables, and whole grains.

Drink 48 to 64 oz of no- or low-calorie fluids throughout the day.

company. Some companies have minimal criteria—for example, a BMI of 35 or greater along with comorbidities or a BMI of 40 or more without comorbidities and a history of inability to achieve durable weight loss.[19] Other companies have rigorous requirements that may include a specified duration of obesity, age limits, drug/alcohol screenings, or participation in medically supervised weight loss programs.[20]

Despite it being a requirement by many insurance providers, there is limited evidence to support mandated preoperative weight loss in order to receive surgical treatment.[7,8] Some insurance companies have acknowledged the lack of evidence while others continue to require a weight loss program; see Box 2.10 on page 43 for examples of insurance requirements.[19,20] Typical programs are 3 to 6 months long with patients monitored by a physician or other health care provider, such as an RDN.

BOX 2.9 Nutrition Care Process Case Study for Preoperative Metabolic and Bariatric Surgery Patient

Nutrition assessment

Patient has a long history of dieting and weight cycling, has type 2 diabetes mellitus, and reports daily intake of six regular sodas. Patient meal and snack patterns are not structured. Patient reports snacking excessively between meals. Patient reports a sedentary lifestyle.

Nutrition diagnosis (PES [problems, etiology, signs and symptoms] statement)

Predicted excessive energy intake related to undesirable food choices of sugar-sweetened beverages as evidenced by intake history of six regular sodas per day.

Nutrition intervention

- Decreased energy diet—reduction in sugar-sweetened beverages
- Modified schedule of foods/fluids—development of structured eating pattern
- Nutrition education content: physical activity guidance
- Nutrition counseling based on:
  - transtheoretical model to stages of change approach
  - motivational interviewing strategy to clarify benefits vs costs of changing
  - cognitive behavioral theory approach to identify substitutes for sugar-sweetened beverages
- Collaboration and referral of nutrition care: referral by nutrition professionals to other providers; referral to exercise physiologist or community program for development of exercise prescription

Nutrition monitoring and evaluation

At follow-up appointment in 2 weeks, evaluate progress with goals. The following outcome indicators are monitored and evaluated:

- Fluid intake: sugar-sweetened beverage estimated oral intake in 24 hours
- Food intake: meal/snack pattern
- Physical activity
  - Consistency
  - Frequency
  - Duration
  - Intensity

BOX 2.10 Sample Insurance Requirements[19,20]

No medical weight loss required

The individual should have documented failure to respond to conservative measures for weight reduction prior to consideration of MBS, and these attempts should be reviewed by the practitioner prior to seeking approval for the surgical procedure. As a result, some centers require active participation in a formal weight reduction program that includes frequent documentation of weight, dietary regimen, and exercise. However, there is a lack of evidence on the optimal timing, intensity, and duration of nonsurgical attempts at weight loss and whether a medical weight loss program immediately preceding surgery improves outcomes.

Medical weight loss required

Documentation of active participation for a total of at least 3 consecutive months in a structured, medically supervised nonsurgical weight reduction program. A comprehensive commercial weight loss program is an acceptable program component, but it must be approved and monitored under the supervision of the health care practitioner providing medical oversight. Comprehensive weight loss programs generally address diet, exercise, and behavior modification (eg, WW or Nutrisystem).

Documentation from the clinical medical records must indicate that the structured medical supervision meets all of the following criteria:

- Occur during a total of at least 3 consecutive months within the 12 months prior to the request for surgery
- Include at least two visits for medical supervision, during the 3 consecutive months of program participation. One visit must occur at the initiation, and another at least 3 months later
- Be provided by an MD, DO, NP, PA, or RDN under the supervision of an MD, DO, NP, or PA
- Include assessment and counseling concerning weight, diet, exercise, and behavior modification

Some insurance providers stipulate that the program include counseling concerning weight, diet, exercise, and behavior modification, but they typically do not specify a therapeutic diet for preoperative bariatric patients.[20] Centers may tailor the preoperative weight loss program based on individual client needs or use a standard weight loss program.

Access to care is a barrier for many people pursuing MBS. The Obesity Action Coalition (OAC) has resources for patients and providers to use when navigating insurance requirements.[20] Box 2.11 contains a list of questions recommended by the OAC when speaking with insurance providers to verify benefits.

BOX 2.11 Questions to Ask When Verifying Benefits[21]

What are your health insurance benefits?

What is the definition of stage III obesity according to your plan?

If any, what coverage of stage III obesity is listed?

What limits or requirements are stated in order to receive stage III obesity treatment? For example:

- Is there a certain amount of required time you must document attempted weight loss?
- Does the documented time have to be consecutive?
- Is your physician required to document your weight loss attempts?
- Do you need to weigh a certain amount before treatment is performed or initiated?
- Is there an age requirement to receive care?
- Must you use a specific Center of Excellence or medical provider to receive coverage?
- Are there weight limitations preventing coverage?

Is there a maximum dollar limit on your benefits?

What treatment options are excluded or specifically included?

What is the copayment for medical services?

What testing is covered, such as nutritionist, psychologist, laboratory, sleep apnea study, and ultrasounds?

Does your insurer require weight loss prior to surgery? If so, what percentage or number of pounds is required?

References

1. Mechanick JI, Apovian C, Brethauer S, et al. Clinical practice guidelines for the perioperative nutrition, metabolic, and nonsurgical support of patients undergoing bariatric procedures—2019 update. *Endocr Pract.* 2019;25(12):1-75. doi:10.4158/GL-2019-0406.GL
2. Sogg S, Lauretti J, West-Smith L. Recommendations for the presurgical psychosocial evaluation of bariatric surgery patients. *Surg Obes Relat Dis.* 2016;12:731-749. doi:10.1016/j.soard.2016.02.008
3. Raynor HA, Champagne CM. Position of the Academy of Nutrition and Dietetics: interventions for the treatment of overweight and obesity in adults. *J Acad Nutr Diet.* 2016;116(1):129-147. doi:10.1016/j.jand.2015.10.031
4. Sherf Dagan S, Goldenshluger A, Globus I, et al. Nutritional recommendations for adult bariatric surgery patients: clinical practice. *Adv Nutr.* 2017;8(2):382-394. doi:10.3945/an.116.014258
5. Parrott J, Frank L, Dilks R, et al. ASMBS integrated health nutritional guidelines for the surgical weight loss patient—2016 update: micronutrients. *Surg Obes Relat Dis.* 2017;13(5):727-741. doi:10.1016/j.soard.2016.12.018
6. Mifflin MD, St. Jeor ST, Hill LA, et al. A new predictive equation for resting energy expenditure in healthy individuals. *Am J Clin Nutr.* 1990;51:241-247. doi:10.1093/ajcn/51.2.241
7. Tewksbury C, Crowley N, Parrott JM, et al. Weight loss prior to bariatric surgery and 30-day mortality, readmission, reoperation, and intervention: an MBSAQIP analysis of 349,016 cases. *Obes Surg.* 2019;29:3622-3628. doi:10.1007/s11695-019-04041-w
8. American Society of Metabolic and Bariatric Surgery. ASMBS updated position statement on insurance mandated preoperative supervised weight loss requirements. ASMBS. April 2016. Accessed May 31, 2020. https://asmbs.org/resources/preoperative-supervised-weight-loss-requirements
9. Busetto L, Dicker D, Azran C, et al. Practical recommendations of the obesity management task force of the European Association for the Study of Obesity for the post-bariatric surgery medical management. *Obes Facts.* 2018;10(6):597-632. doi:10.1159/000481825
10. Colles SL, Dixon JB, Marks P, Strauss BJ, O'Brien PE. Preoperative weight loss with a very-low-energy diet: quantitation of changes in liver and abdominal fat by serial imaging. *Am J Clin Nutr.* 2006;84:304-311. doi:10.1093/ajcn/84.1.304
11. Edholm D, Kullberg J, Haenni A, et al. Preoperative 4-week low-calorie diet reduces liver volume and intrahepatic fat, and facilitates laparoscopic gastric bypass in morbidly obese. *Obes Surg.* 2011;21:345-350. doi:10.1007/s11695-010-0337-2

12. Browning JD, Baker JA, Rogers T, Davis J, Satapato S, Burgess SC. Short-term weight loss and hepatic triglyceride reduction: evidence of a metabolic advantage with dietary carbohydrate restriction. *Am J Clin Nutr.* 2011;93:1048-1052. doi:10.3945/ajcn.110.007674
13. Rubino F, Nathan DM, Eckel RH, et al. Metabolic surgery in the treatment algorithm for type 2 diabetes: a joint statement by international diabetes organizations. *Diabetes Care.* 2016;39(6):861-877. doi:10.2337/dc16-0236
14. Małczak P, Pisarska M, Piotr M, et al. Enhanced recovery after bariatric surgery: systematic review and meta-analysis. *Obes Surg.* 2017;27(1):226-235. doi:10.1007/s11695-016-2438-z
15. Petrick AT, Gadaleta D. Raising the standard: enhanced recovery goals in bariatric surgery (ENERGY): the second MBSAQIP national quality improvement project. Bariatric Times. May 2019. Accessed May 31, 2020. https://bariatrictimes.com/enhanced-recovery-goals-bariatric-surgery
16. Brethauer SA, Petrick A, Grieco A, et al. Employing new enhanced recovery goals for bariatric surgery (ENERGY): a Metabolic and Bariatric Surgery Accreditation and Quality Improvement (MBSAQIP) national quality improvement project. *Surg Obes Relat Dis.* 2018;14(11):S6. doi:10.1016/j.soard.2018.09.021
17. Goldenberg L. Fasting versus carb-loading: what's the evidence for your enhanced recovery after bariatric surgery program? Bariatric Times. November 2018. Accessed May 31, 2020. https://bariatrictimes.com/fasting-versus-carb-loading-whats-the-evidence-for-your-enhanced-recovery-after-bariatric-surgery-program
18. McClave SA, Kozar R, Martindale RG, et al. Summary points and consensus recommendations from the North American Surgical Nutrition Summit. *JPEN J Parenter Enteral Nutr.* 2013;37(5 suppl):99S-105S. doi:10.1177/0148607113495892
19. Highmark commercial medical policy G-24-055—Pennsylvania. Highmark. September 2018. Accessed May 31, 2020. https://securecms.highmark.com/content/medpolicy/en/highmark/pa/commercial/policies/Miscellaneous/G-24/G-24-054.html
20. Medical policy manual—bariatric surgery, policy no. 58. Regence. January 2020. Accessed May 31, 2020. http://blue.regence.com/trgmedpol/surgery/sur58.pdf
21. Access to care resources: helpful tips. Obesity Action Coalition. Date unknown. Accessed May 31, 2020. www.obesityaction.org/action-through-advocacy/access-to-care/access-to-care-resources/helpful-tips

CHAPTER 3

Nutrition Care in the Immediate Postoperative Period

Introduction

Postoperative nutrition care of the metabolic and bariatric surgery (MBS) patient during the first year after surgery has two distinct phases:

- the first 3 months postoperative (the early postoperative phase)
- 3 months to 1 year postoperative

In the early postoperative phase, the registered dietitian nutritionist (RDN) leads the patient through the postoperative diet progression, monitors and helps prevent early nutrition complications, and helps the patient implement a vitamin and mineral supplementation regimen. In the remaining months of the first year, the RDN guides the patient in essential lifestyle and behavior changes to support continuing weight loss. Throughout the year, the RDN's work is guided by the Nutrition Care Process (NCP).

Immediate Postoperative

Enhanced Recovery After Metabolic and Bariatric Surgery

Enhanced recovery (or "fast track") protocols in MBS are designed to reduce length of stay (LOS),[1,2] operation time,[1] readmission rates,[3] and postoperative morbidity,[3] as well as reduce hospital costs.[2] They have been gaining popularity in the MBS community. Preoperative enhanced recovery interventions are discussed in detail in Chapter 2. See Box 3.1 for postoperative enhanced recovery interventions.

BOX 3.1 Postoperative Enhanced Recovery in Metabolic and Bariatric Surgery Interventions[2,4]

Hourly use of incentive spirometry
Fluid balance to avoid fluid overload
Administration of regular multimodal (opioid-sparing) analgesia
Antiemetics
Prokinetics
Laxatives
Early oral intake
Mobilization 2 to 4 hours after returning to hospital unit
Standardized multimodal thrombophylaxis
Early postoperative feeding
Postoperative telephone call

In a randomized clinical trial involving 78 sleeve gastrectomy (SG) patients, LOS was reduced from an average of 2 days to 1 day with enhanced recovery intervention.[2] LOS in SG and Roux-en-Y gastric bypass (RYGB) patients improved by 28% and 37%, respectively. Patients were discharged on postoperative day (POD) 1.[3]

Other enhanced recovery protocols include progression to solid foods with an emphasis on chewing and eating pace 12 hours postoperatively.[4] Bevilacqua and colleagues demonstrated that early feeding reduced LOS from 36.2 to 31 hours, which was statistically significant for primary SG and RYGB cases but not revisional cases. Patients progressed to an MBS-specific full liquid diet on POD 0 instead of POD 1.[5]

Diet 0 to 3 Months After Metabolic and Bariatric Surgery

The postoperative diet in the first 3 months after MBS is typically described in stages. The number of diet stages and recommendations vary among surgical centers. There is no evidence to support a specific protocol of postsurgical diet stages.[6,7] The standardized diet protocol proposed here includes texture progression and considers the fluid, macronutrient, and micronutrient needs of the patient. The diet stages described in the following sections should be adjusted for individual patients as tolerated.[7-10] See Appendix B for more details on the RYGB, SG, biliopancreatic diversion with duodenal switch (BPD/DS), one-anastomosis gastric bypass (OAGB), single-anastomosis duodeno-ileostomy with sleeve (SADI-S), and adjustable gastric banding (AGB) postoperative diet stages and advancement.

Clear Liquid Diet

The first stage in the postoperative diet is a very short-term, clear liquid diet used in the hospital on POD 0 and 1. Note that the hospital LOS for the uncomplicated postoperative patient varies among facilities. The usual stay for patients who have undergone the AGB procedure is one night. For RYGB, SG, and SADI-S patients, the typical stay is two nights.[11-13] Although, some facilities are transitioning to a one-night LOS for SG with the emphasis on enhanced recovery after surgery (ERAS) protocols. Biliopancreatic diversion with duodenal switch patients generally stay two to three nights,[14,15] and OAGB patients stay one night.[16,17] LOS appears to be most influenced by the following characteristics: age (65 and older); diagnoses of chronic obstructive pulmonary disease, hypertension, anemia, or renal insufficiency; BMI greater than 50; and prolonged operative time.[11]

The surgeon may order an upper gastrointestinal (UGI) series to rule out leaks or stricture. Then the patient slowly advances to small sips of clear liquids. These liquids are low in calories and sugar and free of caffeine, carbonation, and alcohol. Warm fluids are often tolerated well after surgery, so encouraging caffeine-free tea and coffee or soup broth can help increase fluid intake. Sugar-free sports drinks can be used for electrolyte support and to encourage fluid intake. Tastes and smell changes are common after surgery, and patients may report an intolerance to water; therefore, flavoring water with sugar-free flavors may increase tolerance.

The RDN should instruct patients to sip liquids in small increments throughout the day, increasing from 1 oz per hour to 8 oz per hour. Using a 1 oz medicine cup can help with sip-pacing. The patient also receives intravenous (IV) hydration, so they should remain well hydrated during this time. However, after discharge, staying hydrated may be a challenge.

Full Liquid Diet

Stage 2 is a full liquid diet. It is started in the hospital or at home after discharge, between POD 0 and 1, depending on the facility. The full liquid diet continues for approximately 10 to 14 days after surgery. In general, many RDNs are moving toward a less conservative diet progression with pureed foods often being introduced before 2 weeks postoperatively to allow for more diet variety. Revisional procedures not impacting the pouch may skip the full liquid phase, instead starting patients on soft foods.

The RDN should give patients lists of specific fluids that meet the stage 2 criteria, such as:

- clear liquids that are caffeine-free, low in sugar and calories, and not carbonated
- full liquids that are low in total and added sugar
    - Fluids should be less than 20 to 25 g total sugar per serving. There is no evidence to support a specific amount of sugar per serving, so recommendations should be tailored to the individual needs of the patient. Patients are advised to avoid added

sugar in the amount advised daily by the American Heart Association (25 g for women and 36 g for men‡).[18]

- Fluids should have 25 to 30 g protein per serving. This includes milk-based beverages, such as fat-free or low-fat milk (or soy or pea protein) mixed with whey, whey-isolate, soy, or other high bioavailable plant-based protein powders. This may include protein-containing clear liquids if milk-based drinks are not well tolerated. Liquids may include commercial protein drinks (premixed or made from powders).

In addition, the RDN should ensure that patients understand how to read food labels in order to:

- limit added sugar, which can lead to dumping syndrome, and
- choose full liquids that meet their daily requirements for protein.

Early postoperative schedules can help a patient meet fluid and protein goals as well as adapt to a long-term eating schedule. The RDN can help the patient develop a time schedule for protein shake or meal replacement consumption, aiming for intake every 3 to 4 hours. The RDN can provide guidance for mealtime schedules to prevent a grazing pattern early on, encouraging the patient to take no more than 30 to 60 minutes to drink a shake.

Recommended Limits on Added and Total Sugars

To prevent dumping syndrome, patients are advised to limit the added sugar content of their protein-containing full liquids. Natural sugars (eg, those found in milk, fruit, and yogurt) are less likely to cause dumping syndrome. There is no evidence to support exactly how much added or total sugar may trigger dumping syndrome in bariatric surgery patients. Therefore, patients should be guided to:

- purchase foods with little to no added sugar and
- limit the total sugar content (from natural and added sugars) to less than 20 g sugar per serving.

These recommendations let patients incorporate foods containing natural sugars, which are an important component of a healthy diet, while minimizing the risk of dumping syndrome.

‡ Data on sex assigned at birth or gender identity was not further specified, and specific recommendations or data for transgender and gender-diverse people were not provided. Please see pages xxi to xxii for more on gender-inclusive terminology.

Evaluating and Selecting Full Liquids to Meet Protein Requirements

During weight loss, consuming smaller servings of protein at each meal may be more metabolically effective than consuming large amounts at one time.[19,20] Therefore, patients should do the following:

- Consume full liquids with more than 15 g protein per serving. In the early postoperative time frame, patients may not finish a complete protein shake, so maximizing protein intake while minimizing volume is ideal.
- Make sure that the protein sources contain the nine essential amino acids.
- Ensure that the full liquids contain some carbohydrates to meet essential needs.

The RDN should review the amino acid composition of the patient's selected protein-containing products.[7] Because of potential limited indispensable amino acids (IAA) from a full liquid diet,[21] the patients are encouraged to consume a variety of protein sources.[7] The protein digestibility–corrected amino acid score (PDCAAS) is one method to evaluate the overall quality and bioavailability of a particular protein product. This impacts the body's ability to use that protein for protein synthesis.[22] The Digestible Indispensable Amino Acid Score (DIAAS), the preferred method of the Food and Agriculture Organization and World Health Organization, along with identifying the IAA,[23] can also be considered. Recommendations for amino acids are as follows:

- Whey, egg white, casein, milk, and soy are types of high-bioavailability proteins recommended for the MBS patient, as they have PDCAAS of 100.
- Collagen and gelatin have low PDCAAS. They lack many essential amino acids and should not be used exclusively postoperatively. However, they may be included in some full liquid products along with other types of protein, such as casein.
- Lysine may be limited in plant-based protein sources.
- Soy protein isolate and pea protein concentrate are limited in methionine and cysteine.

- A plant-based protein powder supplemented with lysine, methionine, cysteine, or other limiting amino acids could be recommended to patients who are following a vegan or vegetarian eating pattern.

In addition to considering the PDCAAS, DIAAS, or IAA, RDNs can evaluate the type of protein and its effect on satiety in the individual patient. Some research suggests that proteins that have a more rapid digestibility, such as whey, have a more satiating effect.[24] Therefore, these types of proteins should be recommended after MBS.

Fluid Goals

To avoid dehydration, the minimum total daily fluid goal is 48 to 64 oz (see Box 3.2). The RDN can teach patients to recognize signs of dehydration and to adjust their clear and full liquid intake accordingly.

Patients who have undergone SG, RYGB, SADI-S, BPD/DS, and OAGB can tolerate only small sips of fluid. They need to be encouraged to sip fluids throughout the day and avoid gulping large volumes of fluid. Patients are encouraged to emphasize fluid intake, even over protein shakes or eating sessions. When patients experience nausea and vomiting related to dehydration, meeting fluid needs becomes increasingly difficult, and IV hydration may be warranted. Dehydration accounts for around 6% of postoperative emergency department visits.[25]

BOX 3.2 Daily Fluid Goals in the Full Liquid Diet

Minimum fluid goal: 48 to 64 oz. Fluid goals are met with clear liquids.

Emphasis should be placed on prioritizing clear liquids over full liquids and protein shakes.

Although some patients may be able to consume the recommended minimum volume on the first day of the full liquid diet, others may need to increase fluid intake in incremental amounts (eg, from one 8-oz serving of full liquids per day to three or four servings per day).

Ensure daily intake of clear liquids is adequate to prevent dehydration. Protein-containing full liquids provide less free water than clear liquids and should never be consumed at the expense of clear liquids.

Patients with the AGB may experience hunger while on the full liquid diet because the band has no saline in it and inflammation from surgery has subsided. During this diet phase, AGB patients are able to tolerate larger volumes of fluid than RYGB, SG, BPD, SADI-S, or OAGB patients. Revisional surgery fluid intake will vary based on procedure and manipulation of pouch size.

Semisolid and Soft Food Texture Progression

These stages begin the process of introducing soft, semisolid foods. Some RDNs may recommend two soft food phases, thus, breaking foods down further by texture. Box 3.3 displays an example of a semisolid diet protocol that includes a soft smooth texture before patients transition to more challenging soft foods. The timing of this stage varies by type of surgery (see Appendix B), and the duration depends on a patient's response to foods.

BOX 3.3 Sample Metabolic and Bariatric Semisolid and Soft Foods

Semisolid foods	*Soft foods*
Greek yogurt without chunks or seeds	Lean ground turkey or chicken
Low-fat cottage cheese	Whole eggs
Low-fat ricotta	Beans or lentils
Fat-free refried beans	Fish
Egg whites or egg beaters	Tuna
Oatmeal, farina, etc	Fork-tender starchy and nonstarchy vegetables
Sugar-free pudding	Low-fat cheese
Canned peaches and pears (packed in water)	
Soft banana	

During the semisolid phase, patients follow a nutrition plan that includes protein, vegetables, fruits, and vitamin and mineral supplements, as well as fluids for hydration. They advance their diet as tolerated, paying attention to physical signals of hunger and satiety. Fruits and vegetables should be introduced and eaten before starches as patients experience early satiety and should prioritize fruits and vegetables.

The RDN should advise patients that regardless of whether they are physically hungry or not, their diet plan is a nutrition prescription at this point and must be followed. Patients should continue to establish an eating pattern that will work for them long term, eating a protein-based food or shake every 3 to 4 hours and adding vegetables, fruits, and whole grains as the volume of their stomach allows. Although stored energy in body fat provides adequate calories, patients need to understand that food and supplements provide essential nutrients. As a patient increases intake of whole protein-based foods, less emphasis can be placed on protein shakes.

In order to make foods more tolerable during the soft foods diet, foods should be cooked using a moist cooking method, such as a crock pot. Low-fat, low-sugar sauces can be added for better tolerance as well. Vegetables and fruits with thick, fibrous, or stringy skins or seeds should be avoided. Slow eating, chewing thoroughly (eg, chewing 20 to 40 times per bite), taking small bites, and mindful eating should be emphasized. Bread, rice, and pasta are often avoided until later diet phases because of their propensity to absorb gastric juices and expand, thus causing stomach discomfort.

Fluid Goals

As semisolid food is introduced, the patient must continue to consume a minimum of 48 to 64 oz of fluids per day. Emphasis on fluid intake vs eating should continue in order to avoid dehydration. After 2 months, fluid volume generally reaches preoperative values, although patients may continue to meet those goals with more frequent drinking intervals.[26]

Introducing Fruits and Vegetables

After a few days of becoming comfortable with what protein foods they can tolerate, the texture of foods, and the rate of eating, patients introduce vegetables and fruits into their diet. Patients should choose nonstarchy vegetables that are well cooked, soft, and moist, and avoid vegetables that are stringy and fibrous. They should also avoid fruits that have skins, seeds, or membranes that could potentially "get stuck."

Introducing Starches

Starches, such as bread, rice, and starchy vegetables, are not recommended in the semisolid stage until the patient is consuming adequate amounts of protein foods, nonstarchy vegetables, and fruits. The fiber in whole grains and the texture of fibrous or stringy vegetables may not be tolerated. Even if they are tolerated, starches are not essential for meeting the patient's nutrient needs at this stage, and eating them may limit intake of more nutrient-dense foods, such as nonstarchy vegetables and fruits.

Mealtime and Postmeal Fluid Recommendations

Traditionally, patients are told to avoid eating and drinking at the same time and are instructed to wait 30 minutes after eating before they resume fluid intake. Drinking with meals may cause dumping syndrome due to the increase in gastric emptying time.[27] Some clinicians also speculate that drinking with meals or within 30 minutes after meals may contribute to weight regain. They theorize that fluids hasten the rate at which solid foods leave the stomach (which would diminish satiety) or add pressure to the new pouch or sleeve, stretching its capacity. The evidence for recommending mealtime or postmeal restrictions on fluid intake to control weight regain are only anecdotal; one study with 28 RYGB patients found patients who ate and drank together consumed more solids, but calorie intake was not significantly greater.[28]

RDNS should *not* routinely advise patients to avoid fluids during the 30 minutes before a meal or snack because there is no evidence that such restrictions are normally beneficial. Liquids typically empty faster than solids and can generally be incorporated up until the mealtime without issue; premeal drinking recommendations can be individualized if needed.

Helping Patients Adhere to the Diet

If patients do not feel hungry, they should still take a few bites of food to stay on their eating schedule. The RDN can encourage patients to stop eating before they feel full, even if food is left on the plate. Leftovers can be saved for the next meal or snack. Box 3.4 on page 58 offers additional tips to help patients tolerate the semisolid diet.

Regular Textures Diet

As weight stabilizes and more foods are tolerated, patients experience increased hunger and are able to eat more food at one sitting. The amount they can eat will vary from meal to meal and from day to day. Patients are advised to continue to plan their meals and snacks and eat mindfully.

In the regular texture phase, patients may slowly add small portions of whole grain foods, such as whole-wheat toast, brown rice, oatmeal, and whole wheat pasta, as well as potatoes and other starchy vegetables, to their meals. However, some foods may cause obstruction or may not be well tolerated. Patients may need to avoid the following:

- untoasted bread
- dry, white poultry
- dry or fibrous meat
- pasta
- rice
- stringy vegetables
- fruits with skins or membranes

Diet 3 Months to 1 Year Postoperative

Once the initial 3 months have passed since surgery, patients are ready to follow a healthy, lifelong diet of nutrient-dense, minimally processed, whole foods to promote weight maintenance. Eating nutrient-dense whole foods helps patients learn to identify the difference between physical hunger and nonphysical hunger cues, which can be more difficult to notice when relying on protein drinks or supplements.

BOX 3.4 Tips for Patients During the Semisolid and Soft Foods Diet

Practice mindful eating.

Take small, dime-size bites.

Chew all food until it is smooth, similar to the consistency of applesauce; then swallow and breathe.

Stop eating as soon as you know the next bite will be too much.

Make sure food, especially meat, is soft and moist enough to swallow without "sticking."

- Marinated meats, boiled meats, and the dark meat of chicken tend to be well tolerated.
- Add chicken broth to dry or fibrous meats (eg, turkey, chicken breast, or hamburger) when reheating them.
- Cooking meat in a slow cooker makes it moist and tender.
- Add low-fat condiments, such as low-fat mayonnaise, mustard, and low-fat gravy, to dry meats.

If food feels "stuck" do not try to push it down by swallowing fluids. Instead, get up and walk around. Drinking fluids will cause more discomfort and possibly regurgitation.

Avoid drinking fluids with meals. It is safe to drink until the time you are ready to eat.

Wait 30 minutes after eating or until your pouch or sleeve is empty to resume drinking.

Follow your nutrition prescription:

- Drink enough for adequate hydration. Needs may vary by person, activity, and season.
- Each day, eat three to five meals or snacks with 1 to 2 oz of protein foods, plus fruits or vegetables.
- Take your vitamin and mineral supplements on schedule.

Avoid bread, rice, and pasta until you can comfortably consume adequate protein, vegetables, and fruits.

Patients should follow a structured meal and snack plan of three meals a day with one or two snacks, if needed. The patient's eating speed and portions must be monitored at this stage to promote weight loss and weight maintenance.

Food intolerance is not uncommon after MBS; prevalence varies by procedure type with the AGB generally reporting the most challenges. Although most MBS surgery types report an increase in tolerance over time, the AGB can cause emerging challenges with subsequent band fills.[29] Foods reported to be most difficult include rice, raw or fibrous vegetables, and chicken or red meat (especially when dry or overcooked). In one study, 31.4% of RYGB patients continued to avoid red meat, 26.4% avoided bread and cereal, and 32.9% avoided milk 2 years postoperatively.[30]

In the early postoperative months, patients are encouraged to wait a few weeks and then retry foods, focus on slow eating, thorough chewing, moist cooking methods, or the addition of a sauce. The MBS patient may continue to struggle to meet fiber needs, even long term. One study reported RYGB patients only consume an average of 11.2 g fiber per day.[31] The RDN should continue to assess for diet quality and food tolerance in order to promote a nutrient-dense, varied diet.

Protein Recommendations

Protein recommendations after MBS aim to minimize the loss of lean body mass. Some evidence suggests that increased protein intake may preserve fat-free mass during weight loss.[24,32] However, exact guidelines for protein consumption have not been defined, and appropriate protein recommendations for individual patients are challenging.[33]

Typical guidelines encourage a minimum of 60 g protein per day[8,32] or up to 1.5 g protein per kilogram of ideal body weight.[8] Even protein distribution with a total of 90 g has been shown to provide a greater 24-hour protein anabolic response compared with unequal distribution,[34] but this research was not conducted in the MBS population. Additional protein may be needed for the highly active patient or those with increased needs related to wound healing, dialysis, or pregnancy.

Patients often focus so much on protein intake that they do not consume adequate carbohydrates or fat. In a typical high-protein diet prescribed for weight loss, an average of 35% of total energy needs is supplied by protein. The RDN can encourage patients to achieve a balanced diet and emphasize the consumption of nonrefined carbohydrates to achieve a protein-sparing effect.

Protein malnutrition is uncommon in uncomplicated bariatric surgery patients but is a risk if oral intake is poor.[7] Refer to Appendix F for more information on preventing and managing protein malnutrition and other complications after MBS.

Alcohol Intake

Alcohol consumption is not advised after MBS. Patients should avoid alcohol for multiple reasons:

- Alcohol is high in calories.
- Tolerance of alcohol is altered after surgery.[35-40]

Weight loss and faster emptying of the gastric pouch contribute to higher blood alcohol content and faster alcohol absorption.[35,37,38]

In addition, patients who have an RYGB procedure experience pharmacokinetic changes that increase alcohol absorption and the time required to eliminate alcohol.[35,37]

Patients with an SG, similar to RYGB, also demonstrate a faster and higher peak blood alcohol level when measured through blood test. Blood alcohol levels appear to be twofold higher than AGB counterparts.[40]

- Alcohol consumption after bariatric surgery may increase the risk of ulcer formation.[41,42]
- Male sex, younger age, smoking, regular alcohol consumption, recreational drug use, lower "belonging" to interpersonal support preoperatively, and having the RYGB are independently related to increased risk of alcohol abuse disorder.[43]
- There is potential for "addiction transfer" (14% to 16% of patients reporting alcohol abuse,[43-45] 7.5% illicit drug use,[43] and 3.5% seeking

substance abuse disorder treatment).[43] The American Society for Metabolic and Bariatric Surgery (ASMBS) advises against alcohol use for at least the first 6 months postoperatively to allow for healing and weight loss[10]; high-risk groups should eliminate alcohol consumption.[8]

Early Postoperative Micronutrient Supplementation

After MBS, patients take vitamin and mineral supplements for the rest of their lives (see Appendix C). Patients begin taking liquid or chewable vitamin and mineral supplements shortly after surgery (typically around the time they start the full liquid diet stage). Patients may eventually progress to supplement tablets if they tolerate and prefer them. Current recommendations suggest waiting 3 to 6 months before progressing to a tablet or capsule form of vitamin,[8,10] but there is no specific literature to support this recommendation.

More research on supplement and medication absorption in MBS patients is needed.[46,47] To support the patient's vitamin/mineral needs, the RDN can provide patients with a list of the essential nutrients to look for in the supplements. A list of over-the-counter products that meet the vitamin and mineral supplementation criteria for MBS patients available locally or online is also useful. The RDN can familiarize themselves with the composition of available products and work with the individual patient to meet their economic, behavioral, and nutrition needs.[48]

Malabsorptive procedures, such as BPD/DS, SADI-S, OAGB, and certain revisional surgeries (ie, limb distalization), will require higher doses of fat-soluble vitamins A, D, E, and K, as well as the minerals zinc and copper. High-dose multivitamins specific for these procedures may be warranted. See Appendix C for more specific vitamin/mineral recommendations.

Rate of Weight Loss in the First 2 Years Postoperative

Weight loss rates vary from patient to patient. Some patients may lose weight at a steady rate each week, whereas others may lose a significant amount of weight intermittently each month. Patients who have an RYGB or SG procedure lose weight rapidly during the first 3 to 6 months after surgery. Initial weight loss for AGB patients is not as rapid. AGB patients may lose weight at a quicker pace after they begin to get band adjustments, which typically occur 4 to 8 weeks after surgery (see Adjustable Gastric Band Adjustments, later in this chapter), and start eating more solid foods. See Table 3.1 for reference on weight loss rates.

The RDN can help support the patient by helping them understand that their particular weight loss rate is unique to them and to instead focus on behavior and lifestyle adjustments. The RDN can help adjust the focus away from the scale and help the patient find success in non-scale victories (NSVs) and changes in health status. Furthermore, patients may expect a steady, smooth rate of weight loss; the RDN can help establish realistic expectations by helping the patient realize postoperative weight loss often has normal periods of short-term plateaus. Patient-centered counseling and shared goal setting can help the patient's needs feel acknowledged and understood; see Appendix H for additional counseling techniques.

Factors that may influence the rate of weight loss among patients having any MBS procedure include the following:

- preoperative weight
- height
- gender
- abdominal fat distribution
- physical activity
- food and beverage choices
- medical status
- medications
- lifecycle stage
- interpersonal support

TABLE 3.1 Weight Loss Rate by Procedure

Procedure	Weight loss outcomes over time							
	1 month	2 months	3 months	6 months	9 months	12 months	18 months	24 months
Adjustable gastric band[49-51]		26% excess weight loss (EWL)		27.2, 30, 45% EWL		38.3, 40% EWL		46.6, 50, 65% EWL
Sleeve gastrectomy[51-53]	18% EWL		31.7% EWL (21.39% total weight loss [TWL])	45% EWL (27.6% TWL)	52% EWL	58.4, 67.7% EWL (30.82% TWL)	64% EWL	64.1% EWL (25.85% TWL)
Roux-en-Y gastric bypass[53,54]			23.87% TWL	32.5% TWL		75.6% EWL (37.7% TWL		78.3% EWL (38.53% TWL)
Biliopancreatic diversion with duodenal switch[55,56ς]				56.9, 61.89% EWL		74.8, 81.49% EWL		
Single-anastomosis duodeno-ileostomy with sleeve[54,57]			17.8%-49% EWL	41%-80% EWL		63.25-95, 83.3% EWL		72-100, 88.6% EWL
One-anastomosis gastric bypass[16]			66.86% EWL	81.05% EWL	83.31% EWL	89.7% EWL	88.4% EWL	88.1% EWL

It is important that patients understand that weight loss occurs in stages, with periods of loss followed by weight plateaus. Because each patient's weight loss pattern is unique, RDNs may want to counsel patients to avoid weighing themselves obsessively or comparing weight losses. The goal is to lose weight in the healthiest manner possible, not as quickly as possible.

Adjustable Gastric Band Adjustments

During the first 4 to 8 weeks after placement of the AGB, patients may feel no restriction because their band is empty. There is little or no saline in the band when it is placed during surgery.

Although uncommon, some AGB patients feel restriction from the adjustable band even when it is not filled. Any restriction felt by a patient with an unfilled band may be caused by residual swelling from the placement of the band.

The first gastric band adjustment typically occurs between 4 and 8 weeks after surgery. Adjustable gastric bands vary in the amount of saline they can hold and the amount of fluid needed to achieve proper restriction. When proper restriction occurs, the patient feels satisfied with smaller portions at meals.

During the first year following adjustable gastric banding, patients should be assessed every 4 to 8 weeks to determine whether the band needs adjustment. The frequency of visits varies among surgical facilities. Weight loss and hunger levels are factors considered in the assessment to determine when subsequent band fills (ie, band adjustments) are needed. Figure E.5 on page 283 provides a tool to assess a patient's hunger. Box 3.5 on page 65 lists signs that indicate the band is too loose or too tight.

Patients reach an optimal stable adjustment level between 1 and 3 years following surgery. After this point, they no longer need regular fills/adjustments. However, as long as the band is in place, all AGB patients should be seen by their surgical team or RDN at least once a year for monitoring of weight, nutritional status, and comorbidity assessment.

After the band is filled, restriction can decrease over time. In addition, patients may experience more food intolerances as the band is tightened, especially regarding breads and dry meats.

BOX 3.5 Adjustable Gastric Banding (AGB) Assessment

Signs a band is too tight

Dysphagia or inability to tolerate solids or liquids

Nighttime cough

Heartburn/reflux/vomiting/sliming

Reliance on soft food intake

Signs a band is too loose

Increased portion sizes

Hunger between meals

Good tolerance of food despite poor eating style ("I can eat anything")

Poor weight loss or weight gain

Patient education should address the complications that can occur following the AGB procedure, such as band slippage, band erosion, port slippage, obstruction, band or tubing leakage, esophageal or pouch dilation, or port leakage (see Appendix F). These complications often require reoperation to correct. If the band is leaking, it will not properly hold the saline needed for restriction. Patients will experience increased hunger and possibly weight gain.

Lifestyle and Behavior Changes

Throughout the first year after MBS surgery, the volume of food that patients can consume increases. Patients may be distressed by their expanding capacity for food, and it is essential to educate them that it is normal. The RDN should encourage them to develop a healthy diet that includes more vegetables, fruits, and whole grains, as well as the protein-rich foods that were the primary focus in the first 3 months after surgery. Patients should also increase their physical activity and participate in structured exercise programs. The RDN can use a variety of counseling techniques (see Appendix H for education and counseling techniques) to help the patient meet lifestyle and behavior change goals.

Nutrition Assessment

First 3 Months After Surgery

Patients routinely have their first formal appointment with the RDN 1 to 3 weeks after MBS. This visit includes a thorough nutrition assessment. Follow-up assessment occurs around 12 weeks after surgery. Refer to Figure E.2 on page 274 for a sample patient questionnaire used at the first postoperative visit. See Figure E.3 on page 276 for assessment data to collect during the follow-up visit at 12 weeks after surgery.

During the first postoperative visit, patients are typically on a semi-solid or soft texture diet. In addition to the information collected using the questionnaire in Figure E.2, the following is information that can be helpful to collect while completing a thorough nutrition assessment (see Box 3.6).

BOX 3.6 Nutrition Assessment for the Immediate Postoperative Metabolic and Bariatric Surgery Patient

Fluid and energy intake

Is the patient consuming adequate fluid intake: volume of clear and full liquids; fluid choices (energy-dense beverages vs low-calorie fluids)?

Is the patient meeting protein intake guidelines?

Are food choices appropriate for the diet stage?

Are the food choices balanced (eg, fiber, fruits, and vegetables) and at appropriate times? Are reported energy levels nonfood related (eg, related to sleep health or stress levels)?

Is the patient consuming whole fruits and vegetables daily?

How frequently is the patient consuming highly processed, low-fiber carbohydrates?

Does the patient have adequate access to safe and healthy food?

BOX 3.6 Nutrition Assessment for the Immediate Postoperative Metabolic and Bariatric Surgery Patient (cont.)

Food tolerance

The following issues related to food tolerances should be assessed at each follow-up visit:

- changes in taste preferences and tolerance of food
- difficulty swallowing
- hunger
- thirst
- lactose intolerance
- sugar alcohol intolerance
- dumping syndrome

Micronutrient intake

Is the patient taking appropriate vitamin and mineral supplements?[a]

- If not, use appropriate counseling techniques to explore the potential challenges (eg, taste, tolerance, access, cost, and remembering).[b]

Does the patient have normal laboratory values?[c]

Does the patient have any signs or symptoms of vitamin or mineral deficiencies?[c]

- See the part on Nutrition-Focused Physical Findings for more information.

Gastrointestinal symptoms

Is the patient experiencing symptoms of dumping syndrome?

Is the patient consuming less than 20 to 25 g total sugar per serving? (Limiting added sugar may help patients avoid dumping syndrome, especially after Roux-en-Y gastric bypass.)

Is the patient experiencing other gastrointestinal (GI) symptoms, such as significant and frequent gas or diarrhea?

Is the patient consuming lactose when these symptoms occur? Does the patient have lactose intolerance?

Is the patient consuming sugar alcohols? (Consumption of sugar alcohols may cause gas and GI upset.)

Continued on next page

BOX 3.6 Nutrition Assessment for the Immediate Postoperative Metabolic and Bariatric Surgery Patient (cont.)

Intake patterns and behaviors

Does the patient consume three to four meals daily, with snacks in between?

Is the patient snacking too frequently throughout the day?

Is the patient allowing for 20 to 30 minutes per meal? Or is the patient eating too quickly and not chewing well?

Does the patient exhibit binge eating patterns or other disordered eating patterns (eg, night eating, grazing, and eating when not physically hungry)?

Is the patient consuming large volumes of liquids with or immediately after meals and snacks?

Physical activity

Is the patient meeting physical activity and exercise recommendations?

Is the patient progressing toward more challenging activities?

Is the patient participating in cardiovascular, resistance, and balance exercises?

Resistance exercises can help promote lean muscle maintenance and reduce bone turnover.

Other topics

What is the patient's level of hunger before meals?

What is the patient's level of fullness after meals?

Is the patient eating in response to nonhunger triggers (eg, locations, emotions, activities, social influence)?

How much food is the patient able to eat at one sitting? Is this amount appropriate for this postoperative period?

How often does the patient participate in moderate to vigorous physical activity?

Does the patient have a positive support system?

Is the patient attending support groups?[d]

BOX 3.6 Nutrition Assessment for the Immediate Postoperative Metabolic and Bariatric Surgery Patient (cont.)

Patient history

Each follow-up visit should include assessment of patient reports of the following:

- diarrhea, constipation, and vomiting
- decreased urination
- fatigue
- medication and supplement use, including changes in types taken, doses, or the administration schedule
- medical/health history—changes in comorbidities or their treatment
- schedule of appointments with surgeon, primary care physician, and other team members

Anthropometric measurements

The assessment at each follow-up visit includes the following anthropometric information about the patient:

- weight
- body mass index
- waist circumference
- amount and rate of weight change
- percentage of excess weight loss

Nutrition-related physical findings

The following data from the physical examination should be noted in the patient's follow-up assessments:

- blood pressure
- heart rate
- condition of skin and mucous membranes (eg, dry skin does not readily return to position after pinching)
- assessment of micronutrient deficiencies
- observation of confusion, concentration changes, motor/gait disturbances, dizziness, or decreased position sense
- understanding of diet stages and guidelines
- amount, type, and duration of physical activity
- patient concerns
- nausea, heartburn, reflux, or dysphagia
- nighttime cough
- abdominal pain and cramping
- stomach grumbling

Continued on next page

BOX 3.6 Nutrition Assessment for the Immediate Postoperative Metabolic and Bariatric Surgery Patient (cont.)

Biochemical surveillance

Laboratory monitoring, including tests to evaluate complete blood count with differential (and hemoglobin A1c for patients with diabetes), which should start 2 to 6 months after metabolic and bariatric surgery

[a] See Appendix C for more information on vitamin and mineral supplements.
[b] See Appendix H for counseling techniques and suggestions.
[c] See Appendix D for more information on laboratory values.
[d] See Chapters 1 and 5 for support group information.

3 Months to 1 Year Postoperative

At 3 months, the patient has likely transitioned to solid, regular textured foods. At each follow-up visit in year 1, the RDN should assess the following:

- meal and snack frequency
- duration of meals
- binge eating patterns and other disordered eating patterns (eg, night eating, grazing, eating when not physically hungry)
- consumption of liquids with or immediately after meals and snacks
- number of meals eaten away from home
- level of hunger before meals
- level of fullness after meals
- nonhunger triggers to eating (eg, locations, emotions, activities, and social influences)
- amount of food patient is able to eat at one sitting
- daily physical activity
- food intolerances
- other food-related issues
- patient history

- anthropometric measurements
- nutrition-related physical findings
- nutrition-related laboratory data

Figure E.4 on page 278 provides a sample nutrition assessment form for an MBS patient more than 6 months postoperatively.

Nutrition Diagnosis

Based on the nutrition assessment, the RDN identifies specific nutrition problems and makes nutrition diagnoses. The nutrition diagnosis is written in a format known as a PES (problem, etiology, and signs and symptoms) statement.[58] Selected nutrition diagnoses that may be applicable in the early postoperative period (0 to 3 months) are provided in Box 3.7; two examples of PES statements are included.

Some post-MBS nutrition diagnoses, etiologies, signs, and symptoms from the first 3 months after surgery continue to apply to patients throughout the first year. Box 3.8 on page 75 features one nutrition diagnosis from this second time period.[58]

BOX 3.7 Selected Nutrition Diagnoses for the Early Postoperative Period (0 to 3 Months After Metabolic and Bariatric Surgery)[a,58]

Inadequate vitamin intake

Sample etiologies	Not taking vitamin supplement Vitamin supplement lacks one or more recommended vitamins
Common signs and symptoms	Reports not taking supplement or taking supplement without all recommended vitamins Physical findings indicative of vitamin deficiency Laboratory findings indicative of low vitamin levels

Inadequate mineral intake

Sample etiologies	Not taking mineral supplement Mineral supplement lacks one or more recommended minerals

Continued on next page

BOX 3.7 Selected Nutrition Diagnoses for the Early Postoperative Period (0 to 3 Months After Metabolic and Bariatric Surgery)[a,58] (cont.)

Inadequate mineral intake (cont.)

Common signs and symptoms
Reports not taking supplement
Reports taking supplement without all recommended minerals
Physical findings indicative of mineral deficiency
Laboratory findings indicative of low mineral values

Sample PES statement
Inadequate mineral (calcium) intake related to not taking calcium supplements, as evidenced by self-report of stopping supplements due to their bad taste.

Undesirable food choices

Sample etiologies
Unwillingness to select food consistent with guidelines
Lack of or change in support systems
Lack of motivation to adhere to guidelines

Common signs and symptoms
Inability, unwillingness, or disinterest in selecting food consistent with guidelines:

- reports consuming solid foods
- reports consuming alcohol
- reports lack of interest or willingness to follow guidelines

Excessive oral intake

Sample etiologies
Unwilling to reduce or uninterested in reducing intake
Food- and nutrition-related knowledge deficit: Adjustable gastric banding (AGB) patients may be unaware that the band may not be "filled" until their first postoperative surgical visit, which may be 4 to 8 weeks after band placement or longer. Although there may be swelling at the band placement site, there is no restriction until the band is filled

Common signs and symptoms
Weight gain not attributed to fluid retention
Reports of intake of:

- foods/beverages with high calorie density
- large portions of food/beverages
- amounts that exceed estimated needs

Binge eating patterns

BOX 3.7 Selected Nutrition Diagnoses for the Early Postoperative Period (0 to 3 Months After Metabolic and Bariatric Surgery)[a,58] (cont.)

Inadequate protein intake

Sample etiologies	Difficulty consuming enough protein due to volume limitations Lack of access to food Economic constraints Food- and nutrition-related knowledge deficit Inappropriate food choices Lack of suppression of gut hormones due to type of procedure (AGB)
Common signs and symptoms	Estimated intake of protein insufficient to meet requirements: • reports of being physically unable to consume enough to meet requirements • not using protein supplements Reports of excessive hunger with AGB

Inadequate fluid intake

Sample etiologies	Inability to consume fluids (nausea, vomiting, or other gastrointestinal [GI] upset/discomfort) Food- and nutrition-related knowledge deficit
Common signs and symptoms	Elevated blood urea nitrogen or serum sodium Dry skin and mucous membranes, poor skin turgor, skin tenting Urine output less than 30 mL/h Reports of: • consuming less than 48 oz total fluid daily • thirst • difficulty swallowing Diarrhea, nausea, vomiting, or GI upset

Continued on next page

BOX 3.7 Selected Nutrition Diagnoses for the Early Postoperative Period (0 to 3 Months After Metabolic and Bariatric Surgery)[a,58] (cont.)

Swallowing difficulty

Sample etiologies	Insufficient chewing of food Eating too much food Eating too rapidly Eating tough foods, doughy bread, overcooked and dry meat Stricture
Common signs and symptoms	Feeling of "food getting stuck" Pain while swallowing Regurgitation

Altered GI function

Sample etiologies	Anastomotic stricture Compromised GI tract function Inability to digest lactose Rapid emptying of sugars and carbohydrates from the gastric pouch into the small intestine, triggering a release of gut peptides Antibiotic use
Common signs and symptoms	Nausea, vomiting, diarrhea, gas, abdominal cramping or pain Constipation Avoidance of specific foods/food groups due to GI symptoms Onset of symptoms associated with the ingestion of simple sugars, lactose, or fried foods
Sample PES statement	Altered GI function related to consumption of milk and apparent lactose intolerance, as evidenced by gas and explosive diarrhea after milk ingestion.

[a] New nutrition-related laboratory tests are not generally done until 8 to 12 weeks after metabolic and bariatric surgery.

BOX 3.8 Example of Nutrition Diagnosis for Patients 3 to 12 Months After Metabolic and Bariatric Surgery[58]

Excessive Energy Intake

Sample etiologies	Food- and nutrition-related knowledge deficit Medications that increase appetite Unwillingness or disinterest in reducing intake Emotional eating
Common signs and symptoms	Weight gain or plateau Intake that exceeds estimated or measured energy needs: • report of increased meal/snack frequency • report of grazing
Sample PES statement	Predicted excessive energy related to indiscrete meal times, as evidenced by diet recall indicating high-calorie foods throughout the day

Nutrition Intervention, Monitoring, and Evaluation

A nutrition intervention defines a plan for changing a nutrition-related behavior, risk factor, environmental condition, or aspect of health status. The goal is to solve the nutrition diagnosis with a two-step process: planning and intervention. Monitoring and evaluation outcome indicators can be used to evaluate the effectiveness of the interventions in the monitoring and evaluation step of the NCP.[58] Box 3.9 features possible nutrition interventions and outcome indicators for nutrition diagnoses made in the first 3 months after MBS. Box 3.10 offers examples of the nutrition interventions and outcome indicators that might be used for a patient in the latter part of the first year who has a nutrition diagnosis of excessive energy intake.

BOX 3.9 Selected Nutrition Interventions and Monitoring and Evaluation Outcome Indicators for Nutrition Diagnoses in the First 3 Months After Metabolic and Bariatric Surgery[58]

Nutrition diagnosis: inadequate fluid intake

Possible interventions

Meals/snacks: increased fluid diet

Food or nutrient delivery: modify schedule of foods/fluid

Monitoring and evaluation outcome indicators

Fluid intake: total fluid estimated intake in 24 hours—amount consumed follows diet stage guidelines

Adherence: nutrition self-monitoring at agreed-upon rate—monitoring fluid intake per hour

Urine profile: urine color—light yellow or clear

Skin: decreased skin turgor—improved or resolved skin turgor

Nutrition diagnosis: swallowing difficulty

Possible interventions

Meals/snacks: modify composition of meals/snacks

- Modify type and amount of foods eaten at meals and snacks—attention to consumption of quantities and food texture per guidelines for diet stage
- Other: eat slowly; set utensil down between swallowed bites

Coordination of nutrition care by a nutrition professional:

- Team meeting involving nutrition professional: communicate all problems identified and planned or recommended interventions to physician and metabolic and bariatric surgery team
- Collaboration with or referral to other providers—including speech pathologist as needed

Monitoring and evaluation outcome indicators

Food intake: amount of food—selection of quantity of foods at meals and snacks per recommendations

Nutrition-focused physical findings: throat and swallowing—reduction or elimination of reports of difficulty swallowing

Nutrition diagnosis: self-monitoring deficit

Possible interventions

Nutrition education content: content-related nutrition education

- Taught use of smartphone application for food tracking
- Reviewed portion sizes vs serving sizes with patient

BOX 3.9 Selected Nutrition Interventions and Monitoring and Evaluation Outcome Indicators for Nutrition Diagnoses in the First 3 Months After Metabolic and Bariatric Surgery[58] (cont.)

Monitoring and evaluation outcome indicators

Adherence: nutrition self-monitoring at agreed-upon rate—tracking food intake for agreed-upon days

Adherence: nutrition self-management as agreed upon—eating based on energy and hunger levels

Adherence: self-reported nutrition adherence score—client assessment of congruence to agreed-upon nutrition-related goal

Nutrition diagnosis: altered gastrointestinal (GI) function: dumping syndrome

Possible interventions

Meals/snacks: modify composition of meals/snacks—limit or omit:

- lactose
- refined sugars
- sugar alcohols
- high-glycemic index carbohydrates
- fats
- fried foods

Modify schedule of food/fluids—ie, foods and fluids are not consumed at the same time

Monitoring and evaluation outcome indicators

Nutrition-focused physical findings: digestive system—reduction or elimination of reports of diarrhea

Nutrition diagnosis: altered GI function: antibiotic-associated diarrhea or* Clostridium difficile *colitis

Possible interventions

Meals and snacks: modify composition of meals/snacks—omit lactose

Nutrition-related medication management: management of nutrition-related prescription management—prescription medication: recommend consideration of initiation of prescription medication to control diarrhea

Nutrition-related medication management: management of nutrition-related over-the-counter (OTC) medication use: complementary/alternative medicine—recommend initiation of probiotics to restore GI tract flora

Continued on next page

BOX 3.9 Selected Nutrition Interventions and Monitoring and Evaluation Outcome Indicators for Nutrition Diagnoses in the First 3 Months After Metabolic and Bariatric Surgery[58] (cont.)

Monitoring and evaluation outcome indicators	Medication and complementary/alternative medicine use: OTC medication use—intake of probiotics per recommendations Nutrition-focused physical findings: digestive system—reduction or elimination of reports of diarrhea

Nutrition diagnosis: altered GI function: constipation

Possible interventions	Increased fluid diet—attention to consumption of fluids per guidelines for diet stage Bioactive substance supplement—psyllium management Increased fiber diet
Monitoring and evaluation outcome indicators	Fluid intake: water estimated oral intake in 24 hours—amount consumed per diet stage guidelines Fiber intake—intake of fiber per recommendations Nutrition-focused physical findings: digestive system—reduction or elimination of reports of constipation

Nutrition diagnosis: altered GI function: malabsorption

Possible interventions	Meals and snacks: increased protein diet—attention to consumption of protein per guidelines for diet stage Vitamin and mineral supplement therapy: • Vitamins supplement therapy—vitamins A, D, E, K • Mineral supplement therapy—calcium (citrated form) and iron (take with vitamin C)
Monitoring and evaluation outcome indicators	Protein intake: measured protein intake—intake of protein per recommendations Measured vitamin intake: vitamin A measured intake over 24 hours—intake of vitamin A per procedure type Estimated mineral intake: estimated calcium intake over 24 hours—intake of specified minerals per recommendations

BOX 3.10 Example of Nutrition Interventions and Monitoring and Evaluation Outcome Indicators for a Nutrition Diagnosis Made More Than 3 Months After Metabolic and Bariatric Surgery[58]

Nutrition diagnosis: predicted excessive energy intake

Possible interventions	Meals and snacks: modify composition of meals/snacks: • low-calorie diet • reduced fat intake • reduced carbohydrate (starch) intake • four to five meals per day, including breakfast • portion control Commercial beverage medical food supplement therapy Increased physical activity
Monitoring and evaluation outcome indicators	Estimated energy intake: total energy estimated intake in 24 hours—decreased by 500 kcal/d per pound of desired weight loss per week Food intake: types of foods—number of food group servings per recommendations Adherence: self-reported nutrition adherence score—good Food intake: amount of food—reduced portion sizes eaten Physical activity: • consistency—increased • frequency—increased • duration—increased • intensity—increased • strength—increased Weight: measured weight—decreased

Nutrition Care Process Case Studies

Boxes 3.11 and 3.12 (see pages 80 and 81) present two case studies illustrating the use of the NCP in the first year after MBS.

BOX 3.11 Nutrition Care Process Case Study for the Early Postoperative Period (0 to 3 Months After Metabolic and Bariatric Surgery)

Nutrition assessment

Patient had adjustable gastric banding and is on full liquids. Patient comes to a follow-up appointment complaining of hunger and reporting intake of a limited amount of protein.

Nutrition diagnosis

Inadequate protein intake related to inappropriate food choices, as evidenced by report of consuming foods with low protein content.

Goals

Protein intake per recommendations

Decreased hunger

Nutrition prescription

60 to 80 g protein per day

Nutrition intervention

Food or nutrient delivery:

- Meals and snacks: modify composition of meals/snacks—modify meals and snacks to include soft, solid protein foods[a]:
    - To prevent or reduce excessive hunger and increase protein intake, start by replacing one full liquid meal with soft, solid protein foods such as eggs and cottage cheese.
    - Increase intake of soft, solid protein foods over next 1 to 2 weeks.
    - Continue to advance diet texture in subsequent weeks.

Nutrition education content:

- Education on nutrition's influence on health
    - Protein's role in satiety
    - Adjustable gastric band's mechanism of action for weight loss

Monitoring and evaluation outcome indicators:

Protein intake: total protein measured intake in 24 hours—meet daily protein goals 5 out of 7 days

[a]Use of very high protein powders and supplements may cause dehydration.

BOX 3.12 Nutrition Care Process Case Study for 6 Months to 1 Year After Metabolic and Bariatric Surgery

Nutrition assessment

Patient status post-sleeve gastrectomy 6 months ago comes for a follow-up appointment. Patient rate of weight loss is less than what was noted at previous appointments, and patient is discouraged by slowing of weight loss.

Nutrition diagnosis

Food- and nutrition-related knowledge deficit related to unrealistic expectations about the pattern of postoperative weight loss, as evidenced by slowing of weight loss and report of discouragement about lack of rapid progress toward weight goal.

Goals

Achievement of realistic expectations about amount and pattern of weight loss

Understanding that total weight is indicative of hydration status as well as fat loss

Use of non-scale measures of success—eg, changes in how clothes fit as an indication of fat loss

Nutrition prescription

Continue energy, vitamin, mineral, protein, and physical activity recommendations.[a]

Nutrition intervention

Nutrition education: content-related nutrition education—including a review of patterns of postsurgical weight loss and reasonable expectations for weight loss amounts

Nutrition counseling: nutrition counseling on cognitive restructuring—reframing success to include nonscale victories

Nutrition monitoring and evaluation

Monitoring and evaluation outcome indicators:

- Beliefs and attitudes: unscientific beliefs/attitudes—increased understanding of expected patterns and amounts of weight and fat loss
- Recommended body weight: goal weight—weight trends and size changes

[a] Registered dietitian nutritionist would state specific amounts

References

1. Wang W, Yang C, Wang B. Meta-analysis on safety of application of enhanced recovery after surgery to laparoscopic bariatric surgery. *Zhonghua Wei Chang Wai Ke Za Zhi.* 2018;21(10):1167-1174.
2. Lemanu DP, Singh PP, Berridge K, et al. Randomized clinical trial of enhanced recovery versus standard care after laparoscopic sleeve gastrectomy. *Br J Surg.* 2013;100:482-489. doi:10.1002/bjs.9026
3. Awad S, Carter S, Purkayastha S, et al. Enhanced recovery after bariatric surgery (ERABS): clinical outcomes from a tertiary referral bariatric centre. *Obes Surg.* 2014;24(5):753-758. doi:10.1007/s11695-013-1151-4
4. Theunissen CMJ, Maring JK, Raeijmaekers NJC, et al. Early postoperative progression to solid foods is safe after Roux-en-Y gastric bypass. *Obes Surg.* 2016;26:296-302. doi:10.1007/s11695-015-1762-z
5. Bevilacqua LA, Obeid NR, Spaniolas K, Bates A, Docimo S Jr, Pryor A. Early postoperative diet after bariatric surgery: impact on length of stay and 30-day events. *Surg Endosc.* 2019;33(8):2475-2478. doi:10.1007/s00464-018-6533-1
6. Academy of Nutrition and Dietetics. Nutrition care in bariatric surgery: diet progression. Evidence Analysis Library. 2008. Accessed May 31, 2020. https://andevidencelibrary.com/topic.cfm?cat=2919
7. Allied Health Sciences Section Ad Hoc Nutrition Committee; Aills L, Blankenship J, Buffington C, Furtado M, Parrott J. ASMBS allied health nutritional guidelines for the surgical weight loss patient. *Surg Obes Relat Dis.* 2008;4(5 suppl):S73-S108. doi:10.1016/j.soard.2008.03.002
8. Mechanick JI, Apovian C, Brethauer S, et al. Clinical practice guidelines for the perioperative nutrition, metabolic, and nonsurgical support of patients undergoing bariatric procedures—2019 update: cosponsored by American Association of Clinical Endocrinologists/American College of Endocrinology, the Obesity Society, American Society for Metabolic & Bariatric Surgery, Obesity Medicine Association, and American Society of Anesthesiologists—Executive Summary. *Endocr Pract.* 2019;25(12):1346-1359. doi:10.4158/GL-2019-0406
9. Mechanick JI, Kushner RF, Sugerman HJ, et al. American Association of Clinical Endocrinologists, the Obesity Society, and American Society for Metabolic & Bariatric Surgery medical guidelines for clinical practice for the perioperative nutritional, metabolic, and nonsurgical support of the bariatric surgery patient. 2008;14(suppl 1):S1-S70. doi:10.4158/EP.14.S1.1

10. Mechanick JI, Kushner RF, Sugerman HJ; for the Writing Group. Executive summary of the recommendations of the American Association of Clinical Endocrinologists, the Obesity Society, and American Society for Metabolic and Bariatric Surgery medical guidelines for clinical practice for the perioperative nutritional, metabolic, and nonsurgical support of the bariatric surgery patient. *Surg Obes Relat Dis.* 2013;9:159-191. doi:10.4158/EP.14.3.318

11. Fletcher R, Deal R, Kubasiak J, Torquati A, Omotosho P. Predictors of increased length of hospital stay following laparoscopic sleeve gastrectomy from the National Surgical Quality Improvement Program. *J Gastrointest Surg.* 2018;22(2):274-278. doi:10.1007/s11605-017-3642-4

12. Carter J, Elliott S, Kaplan J, Lin M, Posselt A, Rogers S. Predictors of hospital stay following laparoscopic gastric bypass: analysis of 9,593 patients from the National Surgical Quality Improvement Program. *Surg Obes Relat Dis.* 2015;11(2):288-294. doi:10.1016/j.soard.2014.05.016

13. Surve AS, Rao R, Cottam D, et al. Early outcomes of primary SADI-S: an Australian experience. *Obes Surg.* 2020;30:1429-1436. doi:10.1007/s11695-019-04312-6

14. Antanavicius G, Sucandy I. Robotically-assisted laparoscopic biliopancreatic diversion with duodenal switch: the utility of the robotic system in bariatric surgery. *J Robot Surg.* 2013;7(3):261-266. doi:10.1007/s11701-012-0372-1

15. Edholm D, Axer S, Hedberg J, Sundbom M. Laparoscopy in duodenal switch: safe and halves length of stay in a nationwide cohort from the Scandinavian Obesity Registry. *Scand J Surg.* 2017;106(3):230-234. doi:10.1177/1457496916673586

16. Carbajo MA, Jimenez JM, Luque-de-Leon E, et al. Evaluation of weight loss indicators and laparoscopic one-anastomosis gastric bypass outcomes. *Sci Rep.* 2018;8(1):1961. doi:10.1038/s41598-018-20303-6

17. Rutledge R, Walsh T. Continued excellent results with the mini-gastric bypass: six-year study in 2,410 patients. *Obes Surg.* 2005;15(9):1304-1308. doi:10.1381/096089205774512663

18. Johnson RK, Appel LJ, Brands M, et al. Dietary sugars intake and cardiovascular health: a scientific statement from the American Heart Association. *Circulation.* 2009;120(11):1011-1020. doi:10.1161/CIRCULATIONAHA.109.192627

19. Millward DJ, Layman DK, Tome D, Schaafsma G. Protein quality assessment: impact of understanding of protein and amino acid needs for optimal health. *Am J Clin Nutr.* 2008;87(5):1576S-1581S. doi:10.1093/ajcn/87.5.1576S

20. Mamerow MM, Mettler JA, English KL, et al. Dietary protein distribution positively influences 24-h muscle protein synthesis in healthy adults. *J Nutr.* 2014;144(6):876-880. doi:10.3945/jn.113.185280

21. Mathai JK, Liu Y, Stein HH. Values for digestible indispensable amino acid scores (DIAAS) for some dairy and plant proteins may better describe protein quality than values calculated using the concept for protein digestibility-corrected amino acid scores (PDCAAS). *Br J Nutr.* 2017;117(4):490-499. doi:10.1017/S0007114517000125
22. Castellanos VH, Litchford MD, Campbell WW. Modular protein supplements and their application to long-term care. *Nutr Clin Pract.* 2006;21:485-504. doi:10.1177/0115426506021005485
23. Rutherfurd SM, Fanning AC, Miller BJ, Moughan PJ. Protein digestibility-corrected amino acid scores and digestible indispensible amino acid scores differentially describe protein quality in growing male rats. *J Nutr.* 2015;145(2):372-379. doi:10.3945/jn.114.195438
24. Faria SL, Faria OP, Buffington C, de Almeida Cardeal M, Ito MK. Dietary protein intake and bariatric surgery: a review. *Obes Surg.* 2011;21(11):1798-1805. doi:10.1007/s11695-011-0441-y
25. Altieri MS, Yang J, Groves D, et al. Sleeve gastrectomy: the first 3 years: evaluation of emergency department visits, readmissions, and reoperations for 14,080 patients in New York State. *Surg Endosc.* 2018;32(3):1209-1214. doi:10.1007/s00464-017-5793-5
26. Dantas RO, Alves LM, Cassiani Rde A, Santos CM. Evaluation of liquid ingestion after bariatric surgery. *Arq Gastroenterol.* 2011;48(1):15-18. doi:10.1590/s0004-28032011000100004
27. Ukleja A. Dumping syndrome: pathophysiology and treatment. *Nutr Clin Pract.* 2005;20:517-525. doi:10.1177/0115426505020005517
28. Arvidsson A, Evertsson I, Ekelund M, Gislason HG, Hedenbro JL. Water with food intake does not influence caloric intake after gastric bypass (GBP): a cross-over trial. *Obes Surg.* 2015;25(2):249-253. doi:10.1007/s11695-014-1401-0
29. Overs SE, Freeman RA, Zarshenas N, Walton KL, Jorgensen JO. Food tolerance and gastrointestinal quality of life following three bariatric procedures: adjustable gastric banding, Roux-en-Y Gastric Bypass, and Sleeve Gastrectomy. *Obes Surg.* 2012;22:536-543. doi:10.1007/s11695-011-0573-0
30. Silver HJ, Torquati A, Jensen GL, Richards WO. Weight, dietary and physical activity behaviors two years after gastric bypass. *Obes Surg.* 2006;16:859-864. doi:10.1381/096089206777822296
31. Novais PFS, Rasera I Jr, de Souza Leite CV, Marin FA, de Oliveira MRM. Food intake in women two years or more after bariatric surgery meets adequate intake requirements. *Nutr Res.* 2012;32(5):335-341. doi:10.1016/j.nutres.2012.03.016
32. Moizé V, Andreu A, Rodríguez L, et al. Protein intake and lean tissue mass retention following bariatric surgery. *Clin Nutr.* 2013;32(4):550-555. doi:10.1016/j.clnu.2012.11.007

33. Moizé VL, Pi-Sunyer X, Mochari H, Vidal J. Nutritional pyramid for post-gastric bypass patients. *Obes Surg.* 2010;20(8):1133-1141. doi:10.1007/s11695-010-0160-9

34. Paddon-Jones D, Rasmussen BB. Dietary protein recommendations and the prevention of sarcopenia. *Curr Opin Clin Nutr Metab Care.* 2009;12(1):86-90. doi:10.1097/MCO.0b013e32831cef8b

35. Klockhoff JC, Naslund I, Jones AW. Faster absorption of ethanol and higher peak concentration in women after gastric bypass surgery. *Br J Clin Pharmacol.* 2002;54(6):587-591. doi:10.1046/j/1365-2125.2002.01698.x

36. Steffen KJ, Engel SG, Pollert GA, Li C, Mitchell JE. Blood alcohol concentrations rise rapidly and dramatically after Roux-en-Y gastric bypass. *Surg Obes Relat Dis.* 2013;9(3):470-473. doi:10.1016/j.soard.2013.02.002

37. Hagedorn JC, Encarnacion B, Brat GA, Morton JM. Does gastric bypass alter alcohol metabolism? *Surg Obes Relat Dis.* 2007;3(5):543-548. doi:10.1016/j.soard.2007.07.003

38. Parikh M, Johnson JM, Ballem N; American Society for Metabolic and Bariatric Surgery Clinical Issues Committee. ASMBS position statement on alcohol use before and after bariatric surgery. *Surg Obes Relat Dis.* 2016;12(2):225-230. doi:10.1016/j.soard.2015.10.085

39. Woodard GA, Downey J, Hernandez-Boussard T, Morton JM. Impaired alcohol metabolism after gastric bypass surgery: a case-crossover trial. *J Am Coll Surg.* 2011;212(2):209-214. doi:10.1016/j.jamcollsurg.2010.09.020

40. Acevedo MB, Eagon JC, Bartholow BD, Klein S, Bucholz KK, Pepino MY. Sleeve gastrectomy surgery: when 2 drinks are converted to 4. *Surg Obes Relat Dis.* 2018;14:277-283. doi:10.1016/j.soard.2017.11.010

41. Dallal RM, Bailey LA. Ulcer disease after gastric bypass surgery. *Surg Obes Relat Dis.* 2006;2(4):455-459. doi:10.1016/j.soard.2006.03.004

42. Sasse KC, Ganser J, Kozar M, et al. Seven cases of gastric perforation in Roux-en-Y gastric bypass patients: what lessons can we learn? *Obes Surg.* 2008;18(5):530-534. doi:10.1007/s11695-007-9335-4

43. King WC, Chen JY, Mitchell JE, et al. Prevalence of alcohol use disorders before and after bariatric surgery. *JAMA.* 2012;307(23):2516-2525. doi:10.1001/jama.2012.6147

44. Reslan S, Saules KK, Greenwald MK, Schuh LM. Substances misuse following Roux-en-Y gastric bypass surgery. *Subst Use Misuse.* 2014;49(4):405-417. doi:10.3109/10826084.2013.841249

45. Spadola CE, Wagner EF, Accornero VH, Vidot DC, de la Cruz-Munoz N, Messiah SE. Alcohol use patterns and alcohol use disorders among young adult, ethnically diverse bariatric surgery patients. *Subst Abus.* 2017;38(1):82-87. doi:10.1080/08897077.2016.1262305

46. Padwal R, Brocks D, Sharma AM. Systematic review of drug absorption following bariatric surgery and its theoretical implications. *Obes Rev.* 2010;11(1):41-50. doi:10.1111/j.1467-789X.2009.00614.x

47. Sawaya RA, Jaffe J, Friedenberg L, Friedenberg FK. Vitamin, mineral, and drug absorption following bariatric surgery. *Curr Drug Metab.* 2012;13(9):1345-1355. doi:10.2174/138920012803341339

48. Majumdar MC, Reardon C, Isom KA, Robinson M. Comparison of bariatric branded chewable multivitamin/multimineral formulation to the 2016 American Society for Metabolic and Bariatric Surgery Integrated Health Nutrition Guidelines. *Obes Surg.* 2020;30:1560-1563. doi:10.1007/s11695-019-04169-9

49. Dargent J. Laparoscopic adjustable gastric banding: lessons from the first 500 patients in a single institution. *Obes Surg.* 1999;9(5):446-452. doi:10.1381/096089299765552729

50. Rubenstein RB. Laparoscopic adjustable gastric banding at a US center with up to 3-year follow-up. *Obes Surg.* 2002;12(3):380-384. doi:10.1381/096089202321087913

51. Belachew M, Belva PH, Desaive C. Long-term results of laparoscopic adjustable gastric banding for the treatment of morbid obesity. *Obes Surg.* 2002;12(4):564-568. doi:10.1381/096089202762252352

52. Sucandy I, Antanavicius G, Bonanni F. Outcome analysis of early laparoscopic sleeve gastrectomy experience. *J Soc Laparoendosc Surg.* 2013;17(4):602-606. doi:10.4293/108680813X13693422520963

53. El Chaar M, Hammoud N, Ezeji G, Claros L, Miletics M, Stoltzfus J. Laparoscopic sleeve gastrectomy versus laparoscopic Roux-en-Y gastric bypass: a single center experience with 2 years follow-up. *Obes Surg.* 2015;25(2):254-262. doi:10.1007/s11695-014-1388-6

54. Enochs P, Bull J, Surve A, et al. Comparative analysis of the single-anastomosis duodenal-ileal bypass with sleeve gastrectomy (SADI-S) to established bariatric procedures: an assessment of 2-year postoperative data illustrating weight loss, type 2 diabetes, and nutritional status in a single US center. *Surg Obes Relat Dis.* 2020;16(1):24-33. doi:10.1016/j.soard.2019.10.008

55. Søvik TT, Taha O, Aasheim ET, et al. Randomized clinical trial of laparoscopic gastric bypass versus laparoscopic duodenal switch for superobesity. *Br J Surg.* 2010;97(2):160-166. doi:10.1002/bjs.6802

56. Praveen Raj P, Kumaravel R, Chandramaliteeswaran C, Rajpandian S, Palanivelu C. Is laparoscopic duodenojejunal bypass with sleeve an effective alternative to Roux en Y gastric bypass in morbidly obese patients: preliminary results of a randomized trial. *Obes Surg.* 2012;22(3):422-426. doi:10.1007/s11695-011-0507-x

57. Shoar S, Poliakin L, Rubenstein R, Saber AA. Single anastomosis duodeno-ileal switch (SADIS): a systematic review of efficacy and safety. *Obes Surg.* 2018;28(1):104-113. doi:10.1007/s11695-017-2838-8

58. Academy of Nutrition and Dietetics. Nutrition Terminology Reference Manual (eNCPT): dietetics language for nutrition care. Accessed June 26, 2020. http://ncpt.webauthor.com

CHAPTER 4

Nutrition Care During Weight Stabilization

Introduction

After metabolic and bariatric surgery (MBS), patients experience periods of weight loss followed by plateaus. Roux-en-Y gastric bypass (RYGB),[1] one-anastomosis gastric bypass (OAGB),[2] and sleeve gastrectomy (SG) patients typically reach their maximum weight loss 12 to 18 months after surgery. The single-anastomosis duodeno-ileostomy with sleeve (SADI-S)[3,4] and biliopancreatic diversion with duodenal switch (BPD/DS) patients have been shown to reach their maximum weight loss 18 months to 2 years after surgery.[4] By 24 months after surgery, most patients experience weight stabilization.[1,3-6]

Once a stable weight is reached, medical nutrition therapy (MNT) focuses on maintenance of a healthy weight, including lifestyle and behavioral changes, and lifelong monitoring of nutritional status. Continued nutrition follow-up in groups or periodic individual appointments with the registered dietitian nutritionist (RDN) can help patients address MBS-related concerns that arise over the long term (see Chapter 1 for an example of standardized postoperative appointments).

Managing Patients' Weight Loss Expectations

An individual patient's total weight loss and rate of weight loss depend on many variables. Outcome data for weight loss by procedure (see Table 1.2 on page 18) can guide expectations, but these data cannot be understood as predictive for any particular individual because they represent averages for a large number of subjects.

The amount/percentage of weight loss varies greatly among patients.[7] Less than 5% of patients lose 100% of their excess body weight, and 10-year postoperative data show weight regain of approximately 20% to 25% from nadir weight is to be expected.[5-9] However, there is less weight regain in BPD/DS patients at 5 years compared with RYGB patients.[10] Psychosocial variables, as well as sedentary lifestyle, poor attendance at postoperative support groups, disordered eating patterns, and poor nutritional food choices may contribute to suboptimal weight loss or weight regain.[11]

Before and after MBS, the RDN should help patients understand that obesity is a chronic and relapsing condition with various etiologies and treatment outcomes. As the patient's rate of weight loss slows and eventually stabilizes, the RDN may need to provide additional education on the stages of weight loss, so the patient does not become discouraged or obsessed leading to other psychosocial issues.

Helping Patients With Weight Maintenance

To succeed with weight maintenance, patients must work to understand their own personal hunger cues, eat mindfully, and stop eating when satisfied. Patients who have had an RYGB, SG, SADI-S, OAGB, or BPD/DS procedure should understand that these metabolic procedures have neurologic and hormonal influences (see Chapter 1), which in turn lead to decreased hunger and increased satiety. Adjustable gastric banding (AGB) is a purely restrictive procedure, and studies have shown that AGB patients, like patients who have lost significant amounts of weight through restrictive dieting, have a higher level of circulating ghrelin. This situation leads to increased hunger.[12]

Visits with the RDN reinforce healthy eating habits as well as lifestyle and behavior changes that promote weight maintenance. Box 4.1 examples guidelines for RDNs working with patients on stabilizing weight. Box 4.2 on page 90 outlines factors that are associated with successful maintenance of weight.[13-17] Chapter 5 focuses on weight regain after MBS.

BOX 4.1 Guidelines for Working With Patients During Weight Stabilization

Educate and involve the primary care physician in the care of postoperative metabolic and bariatric surgery patients, including the following:

- mechanisms of weight loss for each procedure
- weight loss expectations and variables that affect weight loss
- biochemical surveillance of nutritional status[a]
- management of obesity-related comorbidities

Stress the importance of lifelong periodic medical nutrition therapy visits to reinforce healthy eating behaviors.

If a patient experiences significant weight regain, especially in a short period of time, refer them back to the surgeon for assessment of surgical failure or complications of surgery.

[a] See Appendix D for more information.

Nutrition-Related Complications

Adjustable Gastric Banding Complications Requiring Reoperation

The reoperation rate at 12 years post-AGB has been reported in as high as 60% of patients,[18] a factor patients should be made aware of before they select this procedure. Reoperations are primarily due to poor weight loss outcome or complications related to the gastric band. Refer to Appendix F for more complications that may occur with the AGB. Chapter 3 also includes signs that indicate whether a band is too

BOX 4.2 Factors Associated With Successful Postoperative Metabolic and Bariatric Surgery Weight Maintenance[11-15]

Realistic preoperative expectations of weight loss

Adherence to scheduled visits

Compliance with nutrition recommendations

Maintenance of regular physical activity (eg, 150 minutes of moderate or higher intensity physical activity per week)

Periodic assessment to prevent or treat eating or other psychiatric disorders

Participation in support groups

Maintenance of food records and weight monitoring records, when appropriate

Adequate sleep and stress management

Nonfood strategies to cope with emotions and stress

Mindful eating:

- eating slowly
- focusing on the eating experience, without distraction
- paying attention to hunger and fullness

Meal planning

Choosing nutrient-dense whole foods instead of soft, high-calorie foods

Not drinking large amounts of fluids with or immediately after meals

tight/loose. Box 4.3 lists factors that contribute to successful weight loss and weight maintenance after the AGB.[13,17]

Vitamin and Mineral Deficiencies

After MBS, patients must take daily vitamin and mineral supplements for the rest of their lives (see Appendix C). Because the supplementation regimen is demanding and costly, adherence to the regimen often declines over time.[20] Also, patients do not always understand the importance of taking vitamin and mineral supplementation for life in order to prevent deficiencies; therefore, it is important to educate this patient population.[21]

BOX 4.3 Factors Contributing to Successful Weight Loss and Maintenance After the Adjustable Gastric Banding Procedure[13,19]

Frequent band adjustments/fills

Adherence to scheduled visits with the registered dietitian nutritionist and physician

Adherence to post-adjustable gastric band nutrition recommendations:

Planned, structured small meals and snacks:

- Avoidance of high-calorie soft foods
- Avoidance of high-calorie beverages
- Avoidance of drinking while eating and immediately after eating

Micronutrient deficiencies are more likely to develop after the first year of surgery.[7,9,22] See Appendix D for additional information on assessment of laboratory values and common micronutrient deficiencies after MBS.

Reactive Hypoglycemia

Roslin and colleagues[24] suggest that hypoglycemia may contribute to maladaptive eating behaviors and weight regain in some RYGB patients. Reactive hypoglycemia, also called postbariatric hypoglycemia, is most common in RYGB patients because they lack a pyloric sphincter.[23,25] It may also occur in SG and BPD/DS patients, although the mechanism is not as well understood.[26,27] See Chapter 3 for information on the characteristics and prevention of the first phase of dumping syndrome and Chapter 7 for details of the management of postoperative reactive hypoglycemia.

Hair Loss

Human hair follicles have two states: (a) *anagen*, a growth phase, and (b) *telogen*, a dormant or resting stage. Many patients experience early postoperative hair shedding, which is due to telogen effluvium, an alteration in the normal hair cycle that results from emotional or physical stress and is unrelated to protein malnutrition or vitamin and mineral deficiencies.[28] *Hair loss* (alopecia) is more likely to be related to protein malnutrition or deficiencies of certain vitamins or minerals, such as zinc, iron,[29-31] selenium, biotin,[28] and essential fatty acids.[22] See Box 4.4 for reasons to expect a nutritional cause, Appendix G for troubleshooting guidance, and Appendix H for tips on counseling a patient experiencing these challenges.

BOX 4.4 Potential Signs That Hair Loss Is Due to Nutritional Complications of Metabolic and Bariatric Surgery[28-31]

Patients demonstrating any of the following symptoms should be assessed for nutritional deficiencies:

- Hair loss continues more than 1 year after metabolic and bariatric surgery.
- Hair loss starts more than 6 months after surgery.
- Patient exhibits other signs and symptoms of ferritin, zinc, or protein deficiency.

The role of the RDN is to help translate this science of hair loss to patients preoperatively and to help manage expectations when they do lose hair as well as to help evaluate nonscientific approaches and myths perpetuated by other patients pushing specific vitamins or too much protein. The RDN should be able to provide information in order to reduce anxiety about hair loss to patients through counseling interventions.

Role of the Primary Care Physician

Although the incidence of micronutrient deficiencies after MBS increases over time, the number of patients monitored over time significantly decreases.[6-8,22] Patients who do not continue to be followed at the surgical center likely see their primary care physician (PCP) for annual or more frequent appointments. Thus, it is important for the PCP to be educated on the postoperative care of the patient, including weight loss expectations, the importance of adherence to vitamin and mineral supplementation (see Appendix C), biochemical surveillance of markers for nutritional deficiencies (see Appendix D), and management of obesity-related comorbidities. PCPs should also be aware of factors that may contribute to weight regain (see Chapter 5). One role of the RDN is to be proactive in keeping connection with patients and their PCP to help patients maintain continuity of care, regardless of where they go for care. Box 4.5 lists the elements of the PCP's postoperative care for the MBS patient.

BOX 4.5 Essential Elements of Postsurgical Primary Care of the Metabolic and Bariatric Surgery Patient

Monitor for and treat postoperative complications.[a]

Set and encourage realistic weight loss expectations and monitor weight regain.

Manage comorbid conditions—eg, adjust medications for hypertension, dyslipidemia, or diabetes.

Reinforce adherence to vitamin and mineral supplementations.[b]

Ensure required biochemical surveillance.[c].

[a] See Appendix F for more on postoperative complications.
[b] See Appendix C for information on supplementation.
[c] See Appendix D for more on biochemical surveillane.

Comorbid conditions associated with obesity, such as diabetes, hypertension, and dyslipidemia, usually improve after MBS and weight stabilization. The patient's PCP handles the medical management of these comorbidities following surgery. However, it is important to recognize that many patients discuss chronic health conditions more with their RDN, further showing the need for the RDN and collaborative care.

Changes in Health Status

During the first year after MBS, many obesity-related comorbid conditions may resolve or improve (see Box 4.6 on page 94).[7,32-34] The RDN can help discuss changes in health status with the patient, reflecting on successes and nonscale victories (NSVs), independent of weight changes.

BOX 4.6 Improved Comorbidities After Metabolic and Bariatric Surgery

Amenorrhea/infertility
Asthma
Atherosclerotic disease
Cholelithiasis
Degenerative joint disease and restricted mobility
Diabetes
Disordered sleep and sleep apnea
Gastroesophageal reflux
Hyperlipidemia
Hypertension
Infertility
Nonalcoholic steatohepatitis
Obesity-related cardiomyopathy and cardiac dysfunction
Obesity-related hypoventilation syndrome
Osteoarthritis
Polycystic ovary syndrome
Urinary incontinence
Venous stasis disease

Glycemic Control and Type 2 Diabetes

Initial remission of diabetes occurs in 24% to 95% of patients, depending on the definition of remission, the type of surgery, and the type of subjects enrolled in the study.[35] When compared with intense medical therapy, SG and RYGB showed better glycemic control (5% achieved hemoglobin A1c [HbA1c] is less than 6% with medical interventions vs 23% with SG and 29% with RYGB).[36] However, resolution of diabetes is less likely in individuals who have had diabetes for more than 8 years[37] or who are insulin dependent.[34]

Achievement of normal blood glucose levels is more common following RYGB, SG, OAGB, and BPD/DS than AGB.[38] Data from the American College of Surgeons Bariatric Surgery Center Network accreditation program indicated significant improvement of type 2 diabetes at 1 year after surgery in 83% of RYGB patients, 55% of SG patients, and 44% of AGB patients at 109 hospitals.[33] OAGB diabetes remission rates may be as high as 62.5% to 95.9%[34,38] and 95% in BPD.[35]

Patients with type 2 diabetes who have an SG or RYGB procedure and then receive MNT are more likely to achieve a normalized HbA1C level within 1 year of MBS than patients who receive only MNT. Those undergoing RYGB and SG also have a greater reduction in medications for diabetes a year following surgery than patients who receive MNT only.[39]

Weight loss is not the only factor that improves glycemic control in patients who undergo an SG or RYGB procedure. These procedures also affect gut hormones in ways that lead to metabolic changes that contribute to better glycemic control. Resolution or improvement of type 2 diabetes following AGB is exclusively related to weight loss and not related to changes in gut hormones. Refer to Chapter 7 for a discussion of MBS and type 1 diabetes and Chapter 1 for an in-depth review of gut hormones.

Lipid Disorders

Total cholesterol and triglyceride levels may improve (decrease) within 6 months of MBS.[40] High-density lipoprotein (HDL) cholesterol levels gradually increase, with significant improvements by 12 months after surgery.[41] More than 85% of patients have improved triglyceride and HDL levels more than 2 years after surgery.[7]

Sleep Apnea

Mild to moderate sleep apnea may resolve completely after MBS. In a study by Nagendran and colleagues,[37] self-reported sleep apnea remission rates were 60%, whereas Sarkhosh[42] found a 75% improvement in sleep apnea when looking at a systematic review using 13,900 patients; improvement in sleep apnea is demonstrated with all procedures and is not correlated with weight loss.[43] Patients with more severe sleep apnea may continue to have residual apneic episodes[44-46] or have sleep apnea return after an initial remission.[47]

Other Conditions

Obesity hypoventilation syndrome (OHS) may be reduced because intra-abdominal pressure decreases as visceral fat is lost. Sugerman and colleagues [35] found an improvement in arterial blood gases, cardiac dysfunction, lung volume, and sleep apnea index after MBS. There is a 76% rate of remission in OHS following MBS.[7]

Many patients with obesity have hypertension. Foleyand colleagues[48] reported that preoperative hypertension improved in 66% of MBS patients.

Gastroesophageal reflux disease (GERD) is another condition that improves after MBS. Improvement in symptoms of GERD is reported in 70% of RYGB patients, 55% of SG patients, and 64% of AGB patients.[34]

Nutrition Assessment

At each postoperative visit, the RDN collects and evaluates data similar to that collected during the immediate postoperative period (see Chapter 3). See Box 3.6 on pages 69 to 70 and Appendix E for the suggested components of the nutrition assessment.

Anthropometric Measures

At each follow-up visit, the RDN should assess changes in weight and waist circumference/girth. Changes in girth or the size of the patient's clothes can indicate changes in the amount of body fat.

Energy Requirements

Clinicians typically use predictive equations or indirect calorimetry to assess a patient's resting metabolic rate (RMR) and energy requirements. The Mifflin-St. Jeor (for body mass index higher than 30) and Harris Benedict equations are used to estimate RMR; however, neither formula has been validated in patients who have lost significant amounts of weight or had MBS.[49] RDNs should exercise caution when using predictive equations or indirect calorimetry in this patient population, as results may not be accurate.

When using indirect calorimetry, providing appropriate conditions during testing is crucial in obtaining accurate results. These conditions include length of measurement, type of equipment, timing (physical activity, stress, and food), environment of test, and intrasubject variability. Indirect calorimetry can provide a more accurate RMR value when these factors are taken into consideration.[49]

Energy expenditure and, therefore, energy needs vary daily. However, research indicates that bariatric patients can experience an approximate 20% reduction in their RMR up to 2 years postoperatively.[50] Hence, many patients will have a decrease in energy needs after surgery. Patients who graze on food, consume more calories, binge eat, and eat mindlessly have been shown to lose less weight or regain weight after surgery.[51-54] Patients with a history of dieting and weight cycling gravitate toward calorie restriction, which should be avoided after MBS. Therefore, instead of setting calorie limits, the RDN can counsel patients whose weight has stabilized to regulate their energy intake by paying attention to their hunger and satiety and practicing mindful eating and the enjoyment of foods that they choose.[16] Refer to Appendix H for education and counseling techniques. Prioritizing consumption of nutrient-dense foods is important, as MBS patients will have an inability to consume large volumes of food long term. Mindful eating helps ensure not only long-term weight loss success but also a concomitant healthy relationship with food.

Food and Nutrition-Related History

Periodic assessment of food intake helps the RDN identify appropriate interventions to reinforce the importance of healthy food choices and healthy eating behaviors. Patients whose weight has stabilized find that the amount of food they can eat at one sitting has increased. They can typically meet their protein needs and consume three to five servings of vegetables per day. Some patients can incorporate small portions of whole grain foods with some meals.

Biochemical and Medical Surveillance

During the first year after MBS, patients should be tested for vitamin and mineral status. Annual testing is recommended. See Appendix D for more information on the biochemical surveillance schedule.

Nutrition Diagnosis

Selected nutrition diagnoses that apply after year 1 following MBS are listed in Box 4.7. Box 4.8 on page 100 shows an example of a nutrition diagnosis that might occur more than 1 year after surgery.[55] Refer to Chapter 3 for additional examples.

Nutrition Intervention and Nutrition Monitoring and Evaluation

The interventions and outcome indicators for nutrition diagnoses of patients whose weight has stabilized are similar to those for other postoperative time periods. Aside from micronutrient supplementation, the nutrition and behavioral management of the MBS patient is the same as that of a nonsurgical weight management patient. Box 4.9 on page 101 lists nutrition interventions and outcome indicators for the nutrition diagnosis in Box 4.8.[55] See Chapter 3 for additional examples of interventions and indicators that may be relevant in this period.

After the first-year postoperative, patients should have annual visits with the multidisciplinary team, including the RDN. Visits with the RDN for periodic monitoring of weight, intake, and nutrition-related behaviors, even if the patient has no clinically evident complications, may help with healthy long-term weight maintenance.[56]

BOX 4.7 Selected Nutrition Diagnoses for Patients More Than 1 Year After Metabolic and Bariatric Surgery[25]

Inadequate vitamin intake (specify)
Inadequate mineral intake (specify)
Altered nutrition-related laboratory values (specify)
Excessive oral intake
Altered gastrointestinal function
Dumping syndrome (hypoglycemia)[a]
Constipation
Malabsorption
Diarrhea
Lactose intolerance
Self-monitoring deficit
Limited adherence to nutrition-related recommendations
Undesirable food choices
Disordered eating pattern
Unintended weight gain
Physical inactivity
Inability to manage self-care

[a] Used for Roux-en-Y gastric bypass patients.

When patients experience life changes, such as a change in employment, pregnancy, menopause, a change in health or in their support system, they may benefit from additional visits with an RDN or behavioral therapist. These professionals can help the patient find ways to deal with stress or significant emotional problems other than eating.

BOX 4.8 PES[a] for the Nutrition Diagnosis of Inadequate Vitamin Intake (Vitamin B12)[b,7]

Possible etiologies

Not taking vitamin or vitamin B12 supplement

Vitamin supplement lacks recommended vitamin B12

Intolerance of red meat and other foods containing vitamin B12

Common signs and symptoms

Serum vitamin B12 concentration less than 200 to 400 pg/mL

Elevated homocysteine or methylmalonic acid (MMA)

Megaloblastic anemia

Excessive tiredness and fatigue

Tingling and numbness in extremities

Diminished vibratory and position sense

Motor disturbances including gait disturbances

Sample PES statement

Inadequate vitamin B12 intake related to lack of compliance with recommendations for taking additional vitamin B12 supplement with daily multivitamin supplement and intolerance of red meat, as evidenced by reports of fatigue, tingling in extremities, and laboratory signs of low serum vitamin B12 and elevated MMA.

[a] PES = problems, etiology, and signs and symptoms

[b] Due to large body stores of vitamin B12, deficiencies do not often occur within the first 2 years after MBS.

BOX 4.9 Nutrition Interventions and Outcome Indicators for the Nutrition Diagnosis of Inadequate Vitamin Intake (Vitamin B12)[30]

Possible interventions

Meals and snacks: increased vitamin B12 diet

Vitamin and mineral supplements: vitamin supplement therapy—B12

Monitoring and evaluation outcome indicators

Food variety—increased

Food intake: types of food—number of food group servings of vitamin-rich foods per recommendations

Vitamin intake: vitamin B12 measured intake in 24 hours

Self-reported nutrition adherence score—scale of 1 to 10

Nutritional anemia profile: B12, serum

References

1. Sjöström L, Lindroos AK, Peltonen M, et al. Lifestyle, diabetes, and cardiovascular risk factors 10 years after bariatric surgery. *N Engl J Med*. 2004;351(26):2683-2693. doi:10.1056/NEJMoa035622
2. Carbajo MA, Jiminez JM, Luque-de-Leon E, et al. Evaluation of weight loss indicators and laparoscopic one-anastomisis gastric bypass outcomes. *Sci Rep*. 2018;8(1):1961. doi:10.1038/s41598-018-20303-06
3. Enochs P, Bull J, Surve A, et al. Comparative analysis of the single-anastomosis duodenal-ileal bypass with sleeve gastrectomy (SADI-S) to established bariatric procedures: an assessment of 2-year postoperative data illustrating weight loss, type 2 diabetes, and nutritional status in a single US center. *Surg Obes Relat Dis*. 2020;16(1):24-33. doi:10.1016/j.soard.2019.10.008
4. Shoar S, Poliakin L, Rubenstein R, Saber AA. Single anastomosis duodeno-ileal switch (SADIS): a systematic review of efficacy and safety. *Obes Surg*. 2018;28(1):104-113. doi:10.1007/s11695-017-2838-8
5. Sjöström L, Narbro K, Sjöström CD, et al. Effects of bariatric surgery on mortality in Swedish obese subjects. *N Engl J Med*. 2007;357(8):741-752. doi:10.1056/NEJMoa066254
6. Topart P, Becouarn G, Ritz P. Weight loss is more sustained after biliopancreatic diversion with duodenal switch than Roux-en-Y gastric bypass in superobese patients. *Surg Obes Relat Dis*. 2013;9(4):526-530. doi:10.1016/j.soard.2012.02.006

7. Mechanick JI, Kushner RF, Sugerman HJ, et al. American Association of Clinical Endocrinologists, the Obesity Society, and American Society for Metabolic & Bariatric Surgery medical guidelines for clinical practice for the perioperative nutritional, metabolic, and nonsurgical support of the bariatric surgery patient. [published correction appears in *Obesity (Silver Spring)*. 2010 Mar;18(3):649]. *Obesity (Silver Spring)*. 2009;17 suppl 1:S1-70, v. doi:10.1038/oby.2009.28
8. Brolin RE, Gorman RC, Milgrim LM, Kenler HA. Multivitamin prophylaxis in prevention of post-gastric bypass vitamin and mineral deficiencies. *Int J Obes*. 1991;15(10):661-667.
9. Mechanick JI, Youdim A, Jones DB, et al. Clinical practice guidelines for the perioperative nutritional, metabolic, and nonsurgical support of the bariatric surgery patient--2013 update: cosponsored by American Association of Clinical Endocrinologists, the Obesity Society, and American Society for Metabolic & Bariatric Surgery. *Endocr Pract*. 2013;19(2):337-372. doi:10.4158/EP12437.GL
10. Skogar ML, Sundbom M. Weight loss and effect on co-morbidities in the long-term after duodenal switch and gastric bypass: a population-based cohort study. *Surg Obes Relat Dis*. 2020;16(1):17-23. doi:10.1016/j.soard.2019.09.077
11. Sarwer DB, Wadden TA, Moore RH, et al. Preoperative eating behavior, postoperative dietary adherence, and weight loss after gastric bypass surgery. *Surg Obes Relat Dis*. 2008;4(5):640-646. doi:10.1016/j.soard.2008.04.013
12. Mariani LM, Fusco A, Turriziani M, et al. Transient increase of plasma ghrelin after laparoscopic adjustable gastric banding in morbid obesity. *Horm Metab Res*. 2005;37(4):242-245. doi:10.1055/s-2005-861410
13. Pontiroli AE, Fossati A, Vedani P, et al. Post-surgery adherence to scheduled visits and compliance, more than personality disorders, predict outcome of bariatric restrictive surgery in morbidly obese patients. *Obes Surg*. 2007;17(11):1492-1497. doi:10.1007/s11695-008-9428-8
14. Faria SL, de Oliveira Kelly E, Lins RD, Faria OP. Nutritional management of weight regain after bariatric surgery. *Obes Surg*. 2010;20(2):135-139. doi:10.1007/s11695-008-9610-z
15. Evans RK, Bond DS, Wolfe LG, et al. Participation in 150 min/wk of moderate or higher intensity physical activity yields greater weight loss after gastric bypass surgery. *Surg Obes Relat Dis*. 2007;3(5):526-530. doi:10.1016/j.soard.2007.06.002
16. van Hout GC, Verschure SK, van Heck GL. Psychosocial predictors of success following bariatric surgery. *Obes Surg*. 2005;15(4):552-560. doi:10.1381/0960892053723484

17. Orth WS, Madan AK, Taddeucci RJ, Coday M, Tichansky DS. Support group meeting attendance is associated with better weight loss. *Obes Surg*. 2008;18(4):391-394. doi:10.1007/s11695-008-9444-8
18. Himpens J, Cadière GB, Bazi M, Vouche M, Cadière B, Dapri G. Long-term outcomes of laparoscopic adjustable gastric banding. *Arch Surg*. 2011;146(7):802-807. doi:10.1001/archsurg.2011.45
19. Valle E, Luu MB, Autajay K, Francescatti AB, Fogg LF, Myers JA. Frequency of adjustments and weight loss after laparoscopic adjustable gastric banding. *Obes Surg*. 2012;22(12):1880-1883. doi:10.1007/s11695-012-0748-3
20. Cooper PL, Brearley LK, Jamieson AC, Ball MJ. Nutritional consequences of modified vertical gastroplasty in obese subjects. *Int J Obes Relat Metab Disord*. 1999;23(4):382-388. doi:10.1038/sj.ijo.0800830
21. Agaba E, Smith K, Normatov I, et al. Post-gastric bypass vitamin therapy: how compliant are your patients and who is doing the monitoring? *J Obes Bariatrics*. 2015;2(2):5.
22. Allied Health Sciences Section Ad Hoc Nutrition Committee; Aills L, Blankenship J, Buffington C, Furtado M, Parrott J. ASMBS allied health nutritional guidelines for the surgical weight loss patient. *Surg Obes Relat Dis*. 2008;4(5 suppl):S73-S108. doi:10.1016/j.soard.2008.03.002
23. Via MA, Mechanick JI. Nutritional and micronutrient care of bariatric surgery patients: current evidence update. *Curr Obes Rep*. 2017;6(3):286-296. doi:10.1007/s13679-017-0271-x
24. Roslin MS, Oren JH, Polan BN, Damani T, Brauner R, Shah PC. Abnormal glucose tolerance testing after gastric bypass. *Surg Obes Relat Dis*. 2013;9(1):26-31. doi:10.1016/j.soard.2011.11.023
25. Papamargaritis D, Koukoulis G, Sioka E, et al. Dumping symptoms and incidence of hypoglycaemia after provocation test at 6 and 12 months after laparoscopic sleeve gastrectomy. *Obes Surg*. 2012;22(10):1600-1606. doi:10.1007/s11695-012-0711-3
26. Tzovaras G, Papamargaritis D, Sioka E, et al. Symptoms suggestive of dumping syndrome after provocation in patients after laparoscopic sleeve gastrectomy. *Obes Surg*. 2012;22(1):23-28. doi:10.1007/s11695-011-0461-7
27. Hedberg J, Hedenström H, Karlsson FA, Edén-engström B, Sundbom M. Gastric emptying and postprandial PYY response after biliopancreatic diversion with duodenal switch. *Obes Surg*. 2011;21(5):609-615. doi:10.1007/s11695-010-0288-7
28. Halawi A, Abiad F, Abbas O. Bariatric surgery and its effects on the skin and skin diseases. *Obes Surg*. 2013;23(3):408-413. doi:10.1007/s11695-012-0859-x

29. Rojas P, Gosch M, Basfi-fer K, et al. Alopecia en mujeres con obesidad severa y mórbida sometidas a cirugía bariátrica [Alopecia in women with severe and morbid obesity who undergo bariatric surgery]. *Nutr Hosp.* 2011;26(4):856-862. doi:10.1590/S0212-16112011000400028

30. Ruiz-Tovar J, Oller I, Llavero C, et al. Hair loss in females after sleeve gastrectomy: predictive value of serum zinc and iron levels. *Am Surg.* 2014;80(5):466-471.

31. Katsogridaki G, Tzovaras G, Sioka E, et al. Hair loss after laparoscopic sleeve gastrectomy. *Obes Surg.* 2018;28(12):3929-3934. doi:10.1007/s11695-018-3433-3

32. Park CH, Nam SJ, Choi HS, et al. Comparative efficacy of bariatric surgery in the treatment of morbid obesity and diabetes mellitus:a systematic review and network meta-analysis. *Obes Surg.* 2019;19(37):2180-2190. doi:10.1007/s11695-019-03831-6

33. Greenway FL. Surgery for obesity. *Endocrinol Metab Clin North Am.* 1996;25(4):1005-1027. doi:10.1016/s0889-8529(05)70367-4

34. Hutter MM, Schirmer BD, Jones DB, et al. First report from the American College of Surgeons Bariatric Surgery Center Network: laparoscopic sleeve gastrectomy has morbidity and effectiveness positioned between the band and the bypass. *Ann Surg.* 2011;254(3);410-422. doi:10.1097/SLA.0b013e31822c9dac

35. Sugerman HJ, Fairman RP, Sood RK, Engle K, Wolfe L, Kellum JM. Long-term effects of gastric surgery for treating respiratory insufficiency of obesity. *Am J Clin Nutr.* 1992;55(2 suppl):597S-601S. doi:10.1093/ajcn/55.2.597s

36. Schauer PR, Bhatt DL, Kirwan JP, et al. Bariatric surgery versus intensive medical therapy for diabetes—5-year outcomes. *N Eng J Med.* 2017;376:641-651. doi:10.1056/NEJMoa1600869

37. Mechanick JI, Kushner RF, Sugerman HJ; for the Writing Group. Executive summary of the recommendations of the American Association of Clinical Endocrinologists, the Obesity Society, and American Society for Metabolic and Bariatric Surgery medical guidelines for clinical practice for the perioperative nutritional, metabolic, and nonsurgical support of the bariatric surgery patient. *Surg Obes Relat Dis.* 2013;9:159-191.

38. Buchwald H, Avidor Y, Braunwald E, et al. Bariatric surgery: a systematic review and meta-analysis [published correction appears in *JAMA.* 2005 Apr 13;293(14):1728]. *JAMA.* 2004;292(14):1724-1737. doi:10.1001/jama.292.14.1724

39. Schauer PR, Kashyap SR, Wolski K, et al. Bariatric surgery versus intensive medical therapy in obese patients with diabetes. *N Engl J Med.* 2012;366(17):1567-1576. doi:10.1056/NEJMoa1200225

40. Gleysteen JJ. Results of surgery: long-term effects on hyperlipidemia. *Am J Clin Nutr.* 1992;55(2 suppl):591S-593S. doi:10.1093/ajcn/55.2.591s
41. Brolin RE, Bradly LJ, Wilson AC, Cody RP. Lipid risk profile and weight stability after gastric restrictive operations for morbid obesity. *J Gastroenterol Surg.* 2000;4:464-469. doi:10.1016/s1091-255x(00)80087-6
42. Nagendran M, Carlin AM, Bacal D, et al. Self-reported remission of obstructive sleep apnea following bariatric surgery: a cohort study. *Surg Obes Relat Dis.* 2015;11(3):697-703. doi:10.1016/j.soard.2014.10.011
43. Sarkhosh K, Switzer NJ, El-Hadi M, Birch DW, Shi X, Karmali S. The impact of bariatric surgery on obstructive sleep apnea: a systematic review. *Obes Surg.* 2013;23(3):414-423. doi:10.1007/s11695-012-0862-2
44. American Society for Metabolic and Bariatric Surgery. Peri-operative management of obstructive sleep apnea. 2012. Last accessed August 9, 2019. https://asmbs.org/resources/peri-operative-management-of-obstructive-sleep-apnea
45. Sugerman HJ, Kellum JM, Engle KM, et al. Gastric bypass for treating severe obesity. *Am J Clin Nutr.* 1992;55(2 suppl):560S-566S. doi:10.1093/ajcn/55.2.560s
46. Rasheid S, Banasiak M, Gallagher SF, et al. Gastric bypass is an effective treatment for obstructive sleep apnea in patients with clinically significant obesity. *Obes Surg.* 2003;13(1):58-61. doi:10.1381/096089203321136593
47. Fritscher LG, Mottin CC, Canani S, Chatkin JM. Obesity and obstructive sleep apnea-hypopnea syndrome: the impact of bariatric surgery. *Obes Surg.* 2007;17:95-99. doi:10.1007/s11695-007-9012-7
48. Foley EF, Benotti PN, Borlase BC, Holingshead J, Blackburn GL. Impact of gastric restrictive surgery on hypertension in the morbidly obese. *Obes Surg.* 1992;163:294-297. doi:10.1016/0002-9610(92)90005-c
49. Academy of Nutrition and Dietetics Evidence Analysis Library. Energy expenditure: evidence analysis: measuring RMR with indirect calorimetry (IC). Academy of Nutrition and Dietetics. 2006. Accessed June 26, 2020. www.andeal.org/topic.cfm?menu=5299&pcat=2693&cat=2695
50. Academy of Nutrition and Dietetics Evidence Analysis Library. Nutrition care in bariatric surgery: post operative energy needs. Academy of Nutrition and Dietetics. 2017. Accessed July 13, 2020. www.andeal.org/topic.cfm?menu=5308&cat=5614
51. Sorensen KW, Herrington H, Kushner RF. Nutrition and weight regain in the bariatric surgical patient. In: Kushner RF, Still CD, eds. *Nutrition and Bariatric Surgery.* 1st ed. CRC Press; 2015:265-279.

52. Iossa A, Coluzzi I, Giannetta IB, et al. Weight loss and eating pattern 7 years after sleeve gastrectomy: experience of a bariatric center of excellence. *Obes Surg.* 2020;30(10):3747-3752. doi:10.1007/s11695-020-04699-7
53. Chou J, Lee W, Almalki O, et al. Dietary intake and weight changes 5 years after laparoscopic sleeve gastrectomy. *Obes Surg.* 2017;27:3240-3246. doi:10.1007/s11695-017-2765-8
54. Meany G, Conceição E, Mitchell JE. Binge eating, binge eating disorder and loss of control eating: effects on weight outcomes after bariatric surgery. *Eur Eat Disord Rev.* 2014;22(2):87-91. doi:10.1002/erv.2273
55. Academy of Nutrition and Dietetics. Nutrition Terminology Reference Manual (eNCPT): dietetics language for nutrition care. Accessed June 26, 2020. http://ncpt.webauthor.com
56. Endevelt R, Ben-Assuli O, Klain E, Zelber-Sagi S. The role of dietician follow-up in the success of bariatric surgery. *Surg Obes Relat Dis.* 2013;9(6):963-968. doi:10.1016/j.soard.2013.01.006

CHAPTER 5

Inadequate Weight Loss and Weight Regain After Metabolic and Bariatric Surgery

Introduction

Inadequate weight loss and weight regain after any weight management intervention including metabolic and bariatric surgery is possible. However, a distinction should be made between what is inadequate weight loss or abnormal weight regain with that of a usual and expected weight fluctuation. In both surgical and nonsurgical weight loss, the literature defines weight stability and normal weight fluctuation as ±5 kg from nadir (lowest weight).[1,2] Health is not solely defined by weight. One role of the registered dietitian nutritionist (RDN) is to educate patients on a healthy lifestyle that could prevent weight regain. Weight regain could potentially cause relapses in comorbidities, the development of new ones, or the reduction of quality of life. The RDN may also assist the patient in making realistic goals to reaching reasonable weight loss expectations. RDNs should practice a patient-centered approach and focus away from using terms such as "successful" and "unsuccessful" weight loss, as these terms do not denote a personalized nor standardized definition of the many benefits of bariatric and metabolic surgery that transcends merely weight loss.

Anticipated Weight Loss After Bariatric Surgery

Predicting an individual's weight loss or expected weight loss after bariatric surgery is difficult. Longitudinal and meta-analyses indicate the average percentage of excess weight loss (%EWL) differs between MBS procedures, but all procedures provide a durable treatment for obesity.[3] See Box 5.1 for specific data on long-term (more than 10 years) weight loss by procedure.

The durability of weight loss seen with metabolic and bariatric surgery surpasses that of conventional intensive lifestyle intervention. In the seminal National Institutes of Health–sponsored randomized controlled trial called Look AHEAD, the study found only 15% EWL was seen at 8 years.[4] The Look AHEAD intervention focused on including nutrition, physical activity, and behavior modification but not surgery.

Mean %EWL ranges for the most common bariatric procedures show a wide span and are skewed based on the loss to follow-up; therefore, it is difficult to predict with certainty how much weight a patient is expected to lose. A large meta-analysis defined the mean percentage of excess weight loss for all bariatric surgeries to be 61.2% (58.1% to 64.4%) once weight loss stabilized.[5]

Knowing what the research indicates as adequate weight loss ranges after surgery is useful; however, it does not take the place of an individualized approach to patient care. Research shows patients have unrealistic weight loss expectations.[6] The RDN will have a pivotal role in guiding and supporting the patient through their weight loss and health goals.

Inadequate Weight Loss and Weight Regain: Definitions

Controversy continues as to how to best define "successful" weight loss after bariatric surgery and even more debate ensues over what constitutes "inadequate" weight loss. Because bariatric surgery is recognized

BOX 5.1 Long-Term Weight Loss (More Than 10 Years) by Procedure Expressed in Weighed Mean Percent Excess Weight Loss[3]	
Roux-en-Y gastric bypass	55.4%
One anastomosis gastric bypass	80.9%
Adjustable gastric band	45.9%
Biliopancreatic diversion	71.5%
Biliopancreatic diversion with duodenal switch	75.2%
Sleeve gastrectomy	57.0%
Gastroplasty	50.95%

as a metabolic surgery not merely a weight loss surgery, using appropriate terminology is paramount in describing its effectiveness as a treatment option for obesity. Researchers and practitioners alike are deviating from using terms such as "successful" and "unsuccessful" and "failure to lose weight" to describe the status of weight loss after surgery. Terms such as "weight loss responders or nonresponders" and "secondary weight gain" are more properly used terms to describe the situation of weight regain after sugery.[7-9]

However, currently, there are no standardized definitions or metrics used to describe the concept of weight regain and opinions vary. Abnormal weight regain would vary based on the metric used. Body mass index (BMI), %EWL (see Chapter 1 for the calculation of %EWL), percent excess body mass index loss (%EBMIL), and percent total body weight loss (%TWL) are all used interchangeably in the literature. The nadir (lowest weight) of weight loss is reported and observed at 18 months with weight regain beginning and lasting from 24 to 60 months. Definitions currently used in the research literature to describe weight regain are as follows[8-12]:

- BMI increase to 35 or greater after experiencing a BMI of 35 or less
- BMI increase of 5 or more over nadir BMI

Weight Regain

- Any 10 kg increase from nadir weight
- Weight regain of greater than 25% EWL over nadir
- EWL less than 50% after experiencing 50% EWL or more
- Maintenance of total weight loss (TWL) 20% or less

Experts believe that %TWL should be the standard metric used to assess weight loss after MBS since it shows less variability when considering preoperative and predisposing factors that may influence weight loss.[11,12] Research shows a higher preoperative BMI, presence of type 2 diabetes mellitus (T2DM), hypertension, male sex, and age more than 40 years are associated with reduced %TWL in the early postoperative period. Therefore, it is proposed that a weight loss of greater than or equal to 20% TWL defines an efficacious metabolic and bariatric surgery, although this still is not a standardized definition.[12] Until such time a metric and definition can be standardized, RDNs can use these classifications to counsel patients on weight loss expectations and develop lifestyle changes to minimize weight recidivism.

Contributors to Weight Regain

Although MBS is considered a durable and lasting long-term treatment of obesity, the consequence of weight regain is not uncommon, although percentages of how much gained varies among studies, surgical procedure, and the metric used to determine the weight regain. Depending on the surgical procedure and the metric used to denote weight regain, earlier longitudinal studies show that in the RYGB, some weight regain was observed in approximately 50% of the patients. On average, weight gain was 8% from nadir, but this increase in weight did not negate the positive metabolic outcomes of surgery.[13]

Recent data from the Longitudinal Assessment of Bariatric Surgery-2 study showed that the mean weight regain in the RYGB and the AGB between 3 and 7 years was approximately 3.9% and 1.4%, respectively, although patterns of weight regain were variable.[14] Other multicenter longitudinal studies show that at 5 years postoperatively, a mean weight regain of 14.1% of lost weight was seen in populations including RYGB,

SG, and OAGB.[15] In a systematic review of SG, results showed rates of regain ranged from 5.7% at 2 years to 75.6% at 6 years.[16]

There are many contributors to weight regain and secondary weight gain after MBS. Knowing the potential cause will help RDNs in their assessment and interventions to assist patients on resuming and maintaining weight loss. The causes of weight gain are categorized according to the contributing factor (s) and may include the following. More details of each contribution to weight gain are described in Box 5.2 on pages 112 to 113, including the following.

- anatomical surgical changes and complications[16-22]
- physiological, metabolic, and hormonal adaptation[7,16,17,20,23-29]
- comorbid conditions and medications[30,31]
- inadequate lifestyle changes, including dietary and physical activity[2,6,20,31-37]
- psychosocial and behavioral[6,38-44]
- lack of follow-up and support[42,43]

Independent predictors of weight loss and weight regain are shown to be addictive behaviors, depression, and increased maladaptive disordered eating.[44] Patients who are socioeconomically disadvantaged show an association with weight regain after surgery.[45] Race, age, gender (males), having a higher preoperative BMI and a BMI greater than 50, and the presence of comorbid conditions, such as hypertension and T2DM, are also correlated with weight recidivism.[12,46,47] Some studies show that marital status is also an independent predictor of weight regain risk, whereby married patients show a higher risk compared with unmarried.[17]

Prevention and Treatment Options for Weight Regain

Despite the proven long-term efficacy of MBS for weight loss and resolution of comorbid conditions, weight regain continues to be a challenge best treated through an interdisciplinary and intensive

BOX 5.2 Potential Risk Factors for Weight Regain After Bariatric Surgery[2,6,7,16-44]

Anatomical surgical changes and complications[16-22]

Staple line disruption

Stenosis of the pouch outlet

Gastro-gastric fistula

Pouch or stoma dilatation

Poorly constructed bypass or uncalibrated pouch or sleeve

Large volume size of pouch or sleeve

Band slippage or erosion

Physiological, metabolic, and hormonal adaptation[7,16,17,20,23-29]

Changes in resting metabolic rate and energy expenditure

Increases in orexigenic (appetite stimulating) hormones ghrelin and serotonin and decreases in anorexigenic (satiety) hormones (eg, gastric inhibitory polypeptide [GIP], glucagon-like peptide-1 [GLP-1], peptide YY [PYY], cholecystokinin [CCK])

Reactive hypoglycemia

Comorbid conditions and medications[30,31]

Diabetic medications (eg, insulin, thiazolidinediones, sulfonylureas)

Psychiatric and neurologic medications (eg, tricyclic antidepressants, selective serotonin reuptake inhibitors, lithium, antipsychotics, antiseizure, anticonvulsants)

Steroid hormones (eg, oral corticosteroids)

Smoking, alcohol intake, or illegal substance abuse

Inadequate lifestyle changes, including dietary and physical activity[2,6,20,31-37]

Dietary indiscretion and nonadherence to bariatric dietary recommendations

Higher caloric intake

Higher fat and sugar intake

Lower fiber intake

Micronutrient deficiencies

Protein deficiency

BOX 5.2 Potential Risk Factors for Weight Regain After Bariatric Surgery[2,6,7,16-44] (cont.)

Altered food preferences

Sedentary or inadequate energy expenditure

Eating fast food

Eating when feeling full

Weighing oneself less than weekly

Unhealthy dietary and lifestyle practices due to lack of nutritional guidance and knowledge

Food intolerance

Psychosocial and behavioral[6,38-44]

Maladaptive and disordered eating behaviors (eg, nibbling, grazing, night eating, binge eating, loss of inhibitory control)

Depression

Emotional food cravings

Lack of follow-up and support

Unrealistic weight loss expectations

weight loss management program where the RDN is a key member of the team. Reducing the risk of weight regain begins at the start of the weight loss journey with having a patient-centered approach to surgery selection and patient preparation. The surgical treatment for obesity begins with the shared decision between patient and surgeon to choose the most efficacious MBS procedure, followed by patient preparation with a preoperative assessment and education and continued reinforcement of the importance of attending support groups and follow-up care postoperatively.

Postoperatively, continued assessment and education, adherence to dietary guidelines, incorporating physical activity, having support and attending support groups, behavior modification, and continuing follow-up medical care are also paramount in preventing weight regain. See Chapter 4 for more lifestyle and behavioral factors that can promote weight maintenance. This section will describe potential treatment options for weight regain with bariatric surgery. The RDN plays a pivotal role in assessing and educating patients on these treatment options for optimizing positive patient outcomes.

Nutrition and Lifestyle

Weight loss with MBS requires lifestyle changes that the patient must be dedicated to make. One role of the RDN is to facilitate, motivate, and educate patients on what these changes are and help them develop lifelong strategies to maintain weight loss and good health.

A healthy lifestyle after MBS is defined as making sustained changes in food choices and eating behaviors, balancing energy intake with physical activity, adhering to postoperative dietary guidelines including vitamin and mineral supplement intake, participating in support groups, and attending continued follow-up visits with the bariatric team including the RDN.[2,31,36,37,48-51]

Nonsurgical treatment options for patients who have weight regain should include a behavioral and dietary-based medical management program that includes structured dietary intervention.[50] As previously explained, major contributors of weight regain after bariatric surgery are caused by increased energy intake secondary to food choices (fat, sugar, and excess carbohydrates), sedentary activity, and maladaptive eating behaviors; therefore, goals of this program include personalizing and targeting these factors.[49-52]

Research shows a contributing dietary factor that increases energy intake is drinking liquid calories in the form of sugary drinks, liquid supplements, alcohol, and other high-calorie beverages.[51] The RDN can identify these drinking habits and educate patients on more appropriate choices. Another component of a structured dietary intervention includes the addition of portion-controlled meals to reduce energy intake. Although MBS provided the surgical restriction, the RDN can educate on meal planning that can provide nutrient-dense and calorie-controlled meals for satiation, good nutrition, and calorie restriction.[50]

Currently, there are no standardized dietary guidelines for weight regain. A personalized patient-centered approach is best. See Appendix

H for suggested counseling techniques. Researchers have proposed that a diet low in glycemic load that includes a macronutrient breakdown of 45% of carbohydrates, 35% of protein (80 g for women and 100 g for men[‡]), and 20% of fat, with three servings of dairy products, and a supplement of soluble fibers (15 g/d) may be efficacious for resuming weight loss after weight regain.[37] This study, however, included a small sample size of 33 patients who received the Roux-en-Y gastric bypass (RYGB) and who also showed weight regain at more than 2 years after surgery. This macronutrient breakdown should not be considered a guideline for the nutrition management of weight regain, but, rather, it gives the RDN some insight on a dietary intervention that has shown positive outcomes and resumption of weight loss.

Behavioral practices including self-monitoring, continued nutrition follow-up visits, participation in mindfulness approaches to food choices and eating behaviors, and acceptance-based behavioral treatment are all methods of facilitating weight loss.[2,37,44,50-,53] Acceptance-based behavioral therapy targets the root causes of nonadherence to dietary recommendations that have led to weight regain, such as hunger and food cravings that subsequently lead to maladaptive eating behaviors and sabotage weight control.[52] See Box 5.3 on pages 116 to 117 for additional nutrition and behavioral guidelines that help patients maintain weight loss after metabolic and bariatric surgery.

Medications

In 2013, the American Medical Association declared obesity as a chronic disease.[56] Weight loss medications are recognized as an appropriate adjuvant therapy in medical weight management programs. Research shows that weight loss medications can facilitate resumed weight loss in patients with weight recidivism or inadequate weight loss.[57] See Box 5.4 on page 118 for a list of approved weight loss medications.[58] Although RDNs cannot prescribe medications, weight loss medications can be part of their recommendations. In addition, the RDN can assist patients in minimizing nutrition-related side effects that can potentially be seen with these

‡ Data on sex assigned at birth or gender identity was not further specified, and specific recommendations or data for transgender and gender-diverse people were not provided. Please see pages xxi to xxii for more on gender-inclusive terminology.

BOX 5.3 Nutrition and Behavioral Guidelines to Help Patients Maintain Weight Loss After Metabolic and Bariatric Surgery

Basic nutrition and behavioral-related actions to resume weight loss

Follow a balanced meal plan with adequate protein and daily intake of fruit, vegetables, and healthy fats (eg, use MyPlate nutrition guidelines).

Consume at least 48 to 64 oz of fluids each day.

Avoid or minimize intake of high-calorie fluids including regular juices, soft drinks, and other sugar-containing beverages, alcohol, and full-fat dairy.

Adhere to vitamin/mineral supplementation recommendations.[a]

Have nutrition-related laboratory values checked annually.

Eat three meals per day to avoid grazing and nibbling.

Self-monitor food intake, weight, activity, and emotions.

Avoid or minimize concentrated sweets, highly saturated foods, and trans fats.

Eat protein and fiber-containing foods to enhance satiety and feelings of fullness.

Practice mindful eating techniques, such as the following:

- Do not eat in front of the television.
- Chew food well and eat slowly.
- Be aware of physical cues of hunger; avoid drinking fluids with meals. Wait 30 minutes after meals for pouch or sleeve to empty before consuming large volumes of fluids.

Use a small plate (7 to 9 in) to help control portion size.

Consider a diet comprising 45% of carbohydrates, 35% of protein (80 to 100 g), and 20% of fat, with three servings of dairy products, and a supplement of soluble fibers (15 g/d) for weight loss.[37]

Consider prescribing a diet that includes the following[54]:

- 1,200 to 1,800 kcal/d (kilocalorie levels are usually adjusted for the individual's body weight)
- a 500-kcal/d or 750-kcal/d energy deficit if caloric intake assessed as excessive to promote weight loss
- one of the evidence-based diets that restrict certain food types (such as high-carbohydrate foods, low-fiber foods, or high-fat foods) in order to create an energy deficit by reduced food intake

BOX 5.3 Nutrition and Behavioral Guidelines to Help Patients Maintain Weight Loss After Metabolic and Bariatric Surgery (cont.)

Physical activity[55]

Increase activities of daily living, such as walking. Aim for 10,000 steps a day.

Include both resistance training (weight-bearing exercise) and aerobic exercise in the weekly physical activity plan.

- Resistance training strengthens muscles and bones, builds lean body mass, and increases the resting metabolic rate.
- Adults should train each major muscle group 2 or 3 days each week using a variety of exercises and equipment.
- Allow at least 48 hours to pass between resistance training sessions.
- Very light- or light-intensity activities are best for older adults and those who were previously sedentary. Two to four sets of each exercise will help adults improve strength and power.
- For aerobic exercise, aim for 150 to 300 minutes of moderate-intensity activity per week.
- To meet exercise recommendations, engage in 30 to 60 minutes of moderate-intensity exercise 5 days per week or 20 to 60 minutes of vigorous-intensity exercise 3 days per week.
- The desired amount of daily exercise can be achieved in one continuous session or in multiple shorter sessions (of at least 10 minutes). For best adherence and least risk of injury, the duration, frequency, and intensity of exercise should be gradually increased.

Individuals who cannot meet physical activity recommendations can still benefit from some activity. Individuals can consider any of the following:

- walking more around the house
- house chores
- gardening
- leg and arm lifts
- chair exercises

[a] See Appendix C for more information on vitamin and mineral supplementation.

BOX 5.4 Prescription Weight Loss Medications

Medication	*Mechanism of action*	*Side effects and warnings*
Orlistat (Alli)	Reduces fat absorption	Fat-soluble vitamin deficiency, diarrhea, fatty stools, flatulence, stomach pain
Phentermine/ topiramate (Qsymia)	Suppresses appetite	Tingling of extremities, constipation, hypertension, taste changes, teratogenic
Naltrexone/ bupropion (Contrave)	Suppresses appetite	Nausea, constipation, liver damage, hypertension, increased heart rate, suicidal ideation
Liraglutide (Saxenda)	Suppresses appetite and glucose homeostasis	Nausea, vomiting, diarrhea, abdominal pain, increased risk of pancreatitis
Phentermine (Adipex-P, Lomaira, Fastin, Ionamin)	Suppresses appetite	Anxiety, dizziness, hypertension, constipation
Lorcaserin (Belviq, Belviq XR)[a]	Promotes satiety	Headache, dry mouth, fatigue, dizziness, nausea

[a]On January 14, 2020, the Food and Drug Administration had withdrawn lorcaserin from the market citing the results of safety clinical trials showed possible increased risk of cancer. Adapted from the National Institute of Health, National Institute of Diabetes and Digestive and Kidney Diseases. Prescription medications to treat overweight and obesity. Accessed April 22, 2021. www.niddk.nih.gov/health-information/weight-management/prescription-medications-treat-overweight-obesity. See reference 60.

medications. The use of obesity treatment medications is an accepted and recognized practice to treat the disease of obesity and is one of the four pillars of obesity treatment supported by the Obesity Medicine Association (OMA). The other pillars supported by OMA are nutrition, physical activity, and behavior.[59] OMA is the largest professional association of clinicians dedicated to the advancement for the prevention, treatment, and reversal of the obesity disease.

Revisional Surgery

RDNs should be aware that revisional operations, or reoperation secondary to weight regain or relapse of comorbid conditions, may be an option. There are many surgical reoperation techniques including but not limited to converting a sleeve gastrectomy or adjustable band to an RYGB, one-anastomosis gastric bypass, biliopancreatic diversion with or without duodenal switch (considered conversions), endoluminal revision to reduce the size of the stoma, distilizing an RYGB, and many other techniques. However, revisional operations are not recognized as the first course of treatment for weight regain unless there is a medical or surgical complication, such as a fistula or dilatation of the gastric pouch or anastomoses, that instigated the weight regain.[54,61] Not all patients that present with weight regain are candidates for revisional surgery. Results of a full medical, surgical, nutritional, and psychological assessment would determine if the patient is considered for revisional surgery. Risks vs benefits of a reoperation are also assessed, as well as the patient's individual insurance criteria and eligibility for revisional surgery. The RDN, as part of an interdisciplinary team, will continue to assess and educate as though this were a primary procedure. RDNs and all health care providers should have the understanding that the disease of obesity is both chronic and relapsing and recognize that weight regain is not a "fault" but rather a consequence of multifactorial causes. It is of utmost importance for patients to be educated on the revised procedure, as such procedure may be dramatically different in terms of malabsorptive action and may put the patient at increased nutritional risk if not properly assessed and educated.

Nutrition Assessment

Anthropometric Measurements

The 2013 American College of Cardoiology/American Hearth Association Task Force on Practice Guidelines/The Obesity Society Guidelines for the Management of Overweight and Obesity in Adults recommend that a patient's height and weight be measured and the BMI calculated annually. They also recommended that the measurement of waist circumference is also done annually or more frequently patients with overweight and obesity.[62]

Food/Nutrition-Related History

The RDN should note the following about the patient's intake patterns:

- meal and snack frequency
- level of hunger before meals
- level of fullness after meals
- amount of food patient can eat at one sitting
- excessive intake of food in a defined time period
- meals eaten away from home
- place where meal is eaten (kitchen table vs in front of television)
- duration of meals
- mealtime focus (other activities taking place while eating, such as computer work or watching television)
- consumption of liquids at same time as solids
- food textures
- food and beverage choices

Nutrition-Related Physical Findings

The assessment should include patient reports of the following:

- lowest weight achieved
- when weight gain resumed and how much
- nausea, heartburn, reflux, or dysphagia
- nighttime cough
- abdominal pain and cramping
- stomach grumbling

Refer to Appendix E for a sample form to document postsurgical nutrition assessment and other steps in the Nutrition Care Process.

Biomedical Surveillance

Nutrition-related laboratory data should be regularly evaluated in all bariatric procedures (see Appendix D).

Nutrition Diagnosis

Possible nutrition diagnoses during a period of weight regain are listed in Box 4.8 on page 100.

Nutrition Intervention

Nutrition intervention for patients with weight regain after MBS should involve structured dietary invention as part of a comprehensive medical weight management program, as previously discussed. See Box 5.3 on page 117 to review nutrition and behavioral guidelines to help patients maintain or resume weight loss after MBS.

Comprehensive Nutrition Education After Weight Regain

When weight regain occurs in the absence of surgical failure, patients may benefit from more intensive nutrition education and cognitive behavioral therapy. Face-to-face individual sessions, group classes, and online support are all useful. The education process requires much support and repetition on the part of the provider and accountability and practice on the part of the patients. "Back on track" classes for weight regain can help patients make necessary behavioral and lifestyle changes to reverse weight gain or maintain weight loss. All patients should be welcomed without judgment and congratulated for seeking help.

Coordination of Nutrition Care

To ensure the success of patients with MBS, interdisciplinary commitment of health care providers to long-term follow-up care is essential. When the provision of necessary help and support is beyond the scope of RDNs' practice, they should refer patients to an appropriate provider, such as a psychologist or psychiatrist specializing in obesity treatment and weight management. The patient's primary care physician should be involved and educated regarding MBS. RDNs should continue to collaborate with the client's bariatric team as well.

Monitoring and Evaluations

After the first postsurgical year, all MBS patients should have annual visits with the bariatric team, including the RDN. Additional nutrition visits should be scheduled when patients experience weight regain or slip into negative habits. Frequent appointments or nutrition intervention classes may help promote weight loss maintenance or prevention of weight regain. Outcomes of nutrition interventions should be carefully documented.

References

1. Bond DS, Phelan S, Leahey TM, et al. Weight-loss maintenance in weight losers: surgical vs non-surgical methods. *Int J Obes.* 2009;33:173-180. doi:10.1038/ijo.2008.256
2. Stoklossa CJ, Atwal S. Nutrition care for patients with weight regain after bariatric surgery. *Gastroenterol Res Pract.* 2013;2013:256145. doi:10.1155/2013/256145
3. O'Brien PE, Hindle A, Brennan L, et al. Long-term outcomes after bariatric surgery: a systematic review and meta-analysis of weight loss at 10 or more years for all bariatric procedures and a single-centre review of 20-year outcomes after adjustable gastric banding. *Obes Surg.* 2019;29(1):3-14. doi:10.1007/s11695-018-3525-0
4. Pi-Sunyer X. The Look Ahead trial: a review and discussion of its outcomes. *Curr Nutr Rep.* 2014;3(4):387-391. doi:10.1007/s13668-014-0099-x
5. Buchwald H, Avidor Y, Brauwald E, et al. Bariatric surgery: a systematic review and meta-analysis. *JAMA.* 2004;292(14):1724-1737. doi:10.1001/jama.292.14.1724
6. Karmali S, Brar B, Shi X, et al. Weight recidivism post-bariatric surgery: a systematic review. *Obes Surg.* 2013;23:1922-1933. doi:10.1007/s11695-013-1070-4
7. Farias G, Thieme RD, Teixeira LM, et al. Good weight loss responders and poor weight loss responders after roux-en-y gastric bypass: clinical and nutrition profiles. *Nutr Hosp.* 2016;33:1108-1115. doi:10.20960/nh.574
8. Grover BT, Morell MC, Kothari SN, et al. Defining weight loss after bariatric surgery: a call for standardization. *Obes Surg.* 2019;29:3493-3499. doi:10.1007/s11695-019-04022-z
9. Bonouvrie DS, Uittenbogaart M, Luitjen A, et al. Lack of standard definitions of primary and secondary (non) responders after primary gastric bypass and gastric sleeve: a systematic review. *Obes Surg.* 2019;29:691-697. doi:10.1007/s11695-018-3610-4
10. Nedelcu M, Khwaja HA, Rogula TG. Weight regain after bariatric surgery-how should it be defined? *Surg Obes Relat Dis.* 2016;12:1129-1130. doi:10.1016/j.soard.2016.04.028
11. Corcelles R, Boules M, Froylich D, et al. Total weight loss as the outcome measure of choice after roux-en-y gastric bypass. *Obes Surg.* 2016;26:1794-1798. doi:10.1007/s11695-015-2022-y
12. Morell M, Kothari S, Borgert A, et al. Weight recidivism after bariatric surgery. *Surg Obes Relat Dis.* 2017;13(10):S2-S3. doi:10.1016/j.soard.2017.09.009

13. Magro DO, Geloneze B, Delfini R, et al. Long-term weight regain after gastric bypass: a 5-year prospective study. *Obes Surg.* 2008;18:648-651. doi:10.1007/s11695-007-9265-1
14. Courcoulas AP, King WC, Belle SH, et al. Seven-year weight trajectories and health outcomes in the longitudinal assessment of bariatric surgery (LABS) study. *JAMA.* 2018;153(5):427-434. doi:10.1001/jamasurg.2017.5025
15. Baig SJ, Priya P, Mahawar KK, et al. Weight regain after bariatric surgery-a multicenter study of 9617 patients from Indian bariatric surgery outcome reporting group. *Obes Surg.* 2019;29:1583-1592. doi:10.1007/s11695-019-03734-6
16. Lauti M, Kularatna M, Hill AG, et al. Weight regain following sleeve gastrectomy-a systematic review. *Obes Surg.* 2016;26:1326-1334. doi:10.1007/s11695-016-2152-x
17. Maleckas A, Gudaityte R, Petereit R, et al. Weight regain after gastric bypass: etiology and treatment options. *Gland Surg.* 2016;5(6):617-624. doi:10.21037/gs.2016.12.02
18. Yimcharoen P, Heneghan H, Singh M, et al. Endoscopic findings and outcomes of revisional procedures for patients with weight recidivism after gastric bypass. *Surg Endosc.* 2011;25:3345-3352. doi:10.1007/s00464-011-1723-0
19. Heneghan H, Yimcharoen P, BrethauerSA, et al. Influence of pouch and stoma size on weight loss after gastric bypass. *Surg Obes Relat Dis.* 2012;8:408-415. doi:10.1016/j.soard.2011.09.010
20. Alvarez V, Carrasco F, Cuevas A, et al. Mechanisms of long-term regain in patients undergoing sleeve gastrectomy. *Nutrition.* 2016;32:303-308. doi:10.1016/j.nut.2015.08.023
21. Wang X, Lyles MF, You T, et al. Weight regain isrelated to decreases in physical activity during weight loss. *Med Sci Sports Exerc.* 2008;40(10):1781-1788. doi:10.1249/MSS.0b013e31817d8176
22. Reiber BMM, Tenhagen M, Hunfeld MAJM, et al. Calibration of the gastric pouch in laparoscopicroux-en-y gastric bypass: does it matter? The influence on weight loss. *Obes Surg.* 2018;28:3400-3404. doi:10.1007/s11695-018-3352-3
23. Demerdash HM, Sabry AA, Arida EA. Role of serotonin hormone in weight regain after sleeve gastrectomy. *Scand J Clin Lab Invest.* 2018;78(1-2):68-73. doi:10.1080/00365513.2017.1413714
24. Hanvold SE, Vinknes KJ, Bastani NE, et al. Plasma amino acids, adiposity, and weight change after gastric bypass surgery: are amino acids associated with weight regain? *Eur J Nutr.* 2018;57:2629-2637. doi:10.1007/s00394-017-1533-9

25. Santo MA, Riccioppo D, Pajecki, et al. Weight regain after gastric bypass: influence of gut hormones. *Obes Surg.* 2016;26:919-925. doi:10.1007/s11695-015-1908-z

26. Tam CS, Redman LM, Greenway F, et al. Energy metabolic adaptation and cardiometabolic improvements one year after gastric bypass, sleeve gasstrectomy, and gastric band. *J Clin Endocrinol Metab.* 2016;101:3755-3764. doi:10.1210/jc.2016-1814

27. Wolfe BM, Schoeller DA, McCrady-Spitzer SK, et al. Resting metabolic rate, total energy expenditure, and metabolic adaptation 6 months and 24 months after bariatric surgery. *Obesity.* 2018;26:862-868. doi:10.1002/oby.22138

28. Bettini S, Bordigato E, Fabris R, et al. Modifications of resting energy expenditure after sleeve gastrectomy. *Obes Surg.* 2018;28:2481-2486. doi:10.1007/s11695-018-3190-3

29. Pedersen SD. The role of hormonal factors in weight loss and recidivism after bariatric surgery. *Gastroent Res Pract.* 2013;8:528450. doi:10.1155/2013/528450

30. Kyle T, Kuehl B. Prescription medications and weight gain-what you need to know. Obesity Action Coalition. 2013. Accessed February 4, 2021. www.obesityaction.org/community/article-library/prescription-medications-weight-gain/

31. King WC, Belle SH, Hinerman AS, et al. Patient behaviors and characteristics related to weight regain after roux-en-y gastric bypass a multicenter prospective cohort study. *Ann Surg.* 2019. Published online ahead of print. doi:10.1097/SLA.0000000000003281

32. Amundsen T, Strommen M, Martins C. Suboptimal 1316-weight loss and weight regain after gastric bypass surgery-postoperative status of energy intake, eating behavior, physical activity, and psychometrics. *Obes Surg.* 2017;27:1316-1323. doi:10.1007/s11695-016-2475-7

33. Novais PFS, Rasera I, Leite C, et al. Food intake in women two years or more after bariatric surgery meets adequate intake requirements. *Nutr Res.* 2012;32(5):335-341. doi:10.1016/j.nutres.2012.03.016

34. Aron-Wisnewsky J, Verger EO, Bounaix C, et al. Nutritional and protein deficiencies in the short term following both gastric bypass and gastric banding. *PLoS One.* 2016;11(2):e0149588. doi:10.1371/journal.pone.0149588

35. Gero D, Steinert RE, le Roux CW, et al. Do food preferences change after bariatric surgery? *Curr Atheroscler Rep.* 2017;19:38-46. doi:10.1007/s11883-017-0674-x

36. Masood A, Alsheddi L, Alfayadh L, et al. Dietary and lifestylefactors serve as predictors of successful weight loss maintenance postbariatric surgery. *J Obes.* 2019;2019:7295978. doi:10.1155/2019/7295978

37. Faria SL, Kelly EDO, Lins RD, et al. Nutritional management of weight regain after bariatric surgery. *Obes Surg.* 2010;20:135-139. doi:10.1007/s11695-008-9610-z

38. Conceicao E, Mitchell JE, Vaz AR, et al. The presence of maladaptive eating behaviors after bariatric surgery in a cross sectional study: importance of picking or nibbling on weight regain. *Eating Behav.* 2014;15:558-562. doi:10.1016/j.eatbeh.2014.08.010

39. Sarwer DB, Dilks RJ, West-Smith L. Dietary intake and eating behavior after bariatric surgery: threats to weight loss maintenance and strategies for success. *Surg Obes Relat Dis.* 2011;7:644-651. doi:10.1016/j.soard.2011.06.016

40. Hogenkamp PS, Sundbom M, Nilsson VC, et al. Patients lacking sustainable long-term weight loss after gastric bypass surgery shows signs of decreased inhibitory control of prepotent responses. *PLoS One.* 2015;10(3):e0119896. doi:10.1371/journal.pone.0119896

41. Pizato N, Botelho PB, Goncalves VSS, et al. Effect of grazing behavior on weight regain post-bariatric surgery: a systematic review. *Nutrients.* 2017;9:1322-1334. doi:10.3390/nu9121322

42. Vidal P, Ramón JM, Goday A, et al. Lack of adherence to follow-up visits after bariatric surgery: reasons and outcome. *Obes Surg.* 2014;34(2):179-183. doi:10.1007/s11695-013-1094-9

43. Compher CW, Hanlon A, Kang Y, et al. Attendance at clinical visits predicts weight loss after gastric bypass surgery. *Obes Surg.* 2012;22:927-934. doi:10.1007/s11695-011-0577-9

44. Odom J, Zalesin KC, Washington TL, et al. Behavioral predictors of weight regain after bariatric surgery. *Obes Surg.* 2010;20:349-356. doi:10.1007/s11695-009-9895-6

45. Keith CJ, Gullick AA, Feng K, et al. Predictive factors of weight regain following laparoscopic roux-en-y gastric bypass. *Surg Endosc.* 2018;32:2232-2238. doi:10.1007/s00464-017-5913-2

46. Shantavaskinkul PC, Omotosho P, Corsino L, et al. Predictor of weight regain in patients who underwentroux-en-y gastric bypass surgery. *Surg Obes Relat Dis.* 2016;12:1640-1645. doi:10.1016/j.soard.2016.08.028

47. Lufti R, Torquati A, Sekhar N, et al. Predictors of success after laparoscopic gastric bypass: a multivariate analysis of socioeconomic factors. *Surg Endosc.* 2006;20:864-867. doi:10.1007/s00464-005-0115-8

48. Kalarchian MA, Marcus MD, Courcoulas AP, et al. Optimizing long-term weight control after bariatric surgery: a pilot study. *Surg Obes Relat Dis.* 2012;8:710-716.

49. Srivastava G, Buffington C. A specialized medical management program to address post-operative weight regain in bariatric patients. *Obes Surg.* 2018;28:2241-2246. doi:10.1007/s11695-018-3141-z

50. Kalarchian MA, Marcus MD, Courcoulas AP, et al. Structured dietary intervention to facilitate weight loss after bariatric surgery: a randomized, controlled pilot study. *Obesity.* 2016;24:1906-1912. doi:10.1002/oby.21591
51. McGrice M, Paul KD. Interventions to improve long-term weight loss in patients following bariatric surgery: challenges and solutions. *Diabetes Metab Syndr Obes Targets Ther.* 2015;8:263-274. doi:10.2147/DMSO.S57054
52. Bradley LE, Forman EM, Kerrigan SG, et al. A pilot study of an acceptance-based behavioral intervention for weight regain after bariatric surgery. *Obes Surg.* 2016;26:2433-2441. doi:10.1007/s11695-016-2125-0
53. Chacko SA, Yeh GY, Davis RB, et al. A mindfulness-based intervention to control weight after bariatric surgery: preliminary results from a randomized controlled pilot trail. *Complement Ther Med.* 2016;28:13-21. doi:10.1016/j.ctim.2016.07.001
54. Dakin GF, Eid G, Mikami D, et al. Endoluminal revision of gastric bypass for weight regain-a systematic review. *Surg Obes Relat Dis.* 2013;9:335-343. doi:10.1016/j.soard.2013.03.001
55. Physical activity guidelines for Americans. February 2019. US. Department of Health and Human Services. Accessed March 14, 2021. https://health.gov/sites/default/files/2019-09/Physical_Activity_Guidelines_2nd_edition.pdf
56. Obesity. American Medical Association. 1995-2020. Accessed February 20, 2020. www.ama-assn.org/search?search=obesity+disease
57. Stranford FC, Alfaris N, Gomez, G, et al. The utility of weight loss medications after bariatric surgery for weight regain or inadequate weight loss: a multi-center study. *Surg Obes Relat Dis.* 2017;13(3):491-500. doi:10.1016/j.soard.2016.10.018
58. Prescription medications to treat overweight and obesity. 2019-2020. NIH National Institute of Diabetes and Digestive and Kidnesy Disease. Accessed February 20, 2020. www.niddk.nih.gov/health-information/weight-management/prescription-medications-treat-overweight-obesity
59. Obesity Medicine Association. About OMA. Accessed December 20, 2020. https://obesitymedicine.org/about/about-oma
60. National Institute of Health, National Institute of Diabetes and Digestive and Kidney Diseases. Prescription medications to treat overweight and obesity. Accessed April 22, 2022. www.niddk.nih.gov/health-information/weight-management/prescription-medications-treat-overweight-obesity

61. Cambi MPC, Marchesini SD, Baretta GAP. Post bariatric surgery weight regain: evaluation of nutritional profile of candidate patients for endoscopic argon plasma coagulation. *ABCD Arq Bras Cir Dig.* 2015;28(1):40-43. doi:10.1590/S0102-6720201500010001

62. Jensen MD, Ryen DH, Apovian CM, et al. 2013 AHA/ACC/TOS guideline for the management of overweight and obesity in adults: a report of the American College of Cardiology/American Heart Association Task Force on practice guidelines and the Obesity Society. *Circulation.* 2014;63:2985-3023.

CHAPTER 6

Metabolic and Bariatric Surgery in Adolescents

Introduction

The prevalence of obesity in US adolescents is approaching 20%. Between 1999–2000 and 2016 National Health and Nutrition Examination Survey (NHANES), the prevalence of obesity and severe obesity in adolescents steadily and significantly increased.[1] Adolescents with severe obesity have increased risk of comorbidities, including obstructive sleep apnea, diabetes, hypertension, dyslipidemia, hyperinsulinism, and depression, along with decreased quality of life.[2-4]

In adolescent patients, noninvasive approaches to weight loss that use behavioral, multidisciplinary, family-based techniques are preferable. However, data suggest that these approaches rarely lead to long-term successful weight loss in adolescents with severe obesity.[5] Data analyzing weight loss after metabolic and bariatric surgery (MBS) demonstrate a sustained decrease in body mass index (BMI), establishing this approach as an effective intervention for severe obesity in adolescents.[6-12] Adolescent MBS can also help improve or resolve severe comorbid conditions associated with obesity in adolescents, such as type 2 diabetes, obstructive sleep apnea, benign intracranial hypertension, nonalcoholic steatohepatitis, hypertension, and cardiovascular risk factors.[6-13]

In 2019, the American Academy of Pediatrics (AAP) issued a statement recognizing the role MBS treatment can play for qualified adolescents (age 13 to 18 years) with severe obesity.[14] AAP also advocates for adolescents with severe obesity of all racial, ethnic, and socioeconomic backgrounds to have access to high-quality multidisciplinary pediatric MBS programs.[14]

Adolescent MBS seems to have the same risks and benefits as MBS in adults.[15,16] For example, two retrospective studies evaluating adolescent MBS trends found complication rates as low as those seen in adults undergoing MBS procedures.[8,16]

Studies have provided a number of evidence-based and best practice guidelines for adolescent MBS.[17-24] The most common procedures performed in adolescents are sleeve gastrectomy (SG) and Roux-en-Y gastric bypass (RYGB).[12] Both procedures have been shown to provide clinically significant and durable weight loss in adolescents with severe obesity. A meta-analysis of 37 studies in adolescents undergoing MBS compared efficacy and health benefits of the RYGB, SG, and adjustable gastric band (AGB).[11] A mean BMI loss of 16.6 after RYBG and a loss of 14.1 after SG was reported.[11]

The PCORnet Bariatric Study of adolescents undergoing MBS in the United States reported similar findings. Analyses of that data set found that at 1-year follow-up, mean BMI changes were −31% for RYGB and −28% for SG. At 3 years, mean BMI changes were −29% for RYGB and −25% for those undergoing SG. At 5 years, data were insufficient to make statistical comparison between the two procedures. However, the authors noted trends toward stabilization of BMI in both RYGB and SG was evident.[12] Overall, adolescents undergoing RYGB and SG experienced similar declines in BMI.

As previously stated, MBS provided marked improvements in most obesity-related health concerns in adolescents. Selection of MBS procedure type for adolescents should be discussed with the medical provider to determine the potential impact of MBS on BMI and health outcomes as well as the impact on long-term health maintenance factors when determining which surgery type to select for the adolescent considering metabolic and MBS.

Preoperative Evaluation

Institutions should provide MBS to adolescents only if a multidisciplinary team dedicated to providing both preoperative and postoperative care to this unique population is in place to ensure safety and excellent delivery of clinical care. Ideally, a registered dietitian nutritionist (RDN) with a certificate in pediatric/adult weight management, such as the Commission on Dietetic Registration's (CDR's) Certificate of Training in Obesity in Pediatrics and Adults, CDR's designation of Certified Specialist in Obesity and Weight Management (CSOWM), or experience in MBS will evaluate and monitor the nutritional status of the adolescent undergoing MBS and provide education throughout the process.[24,25] Other members of the multidisciplinary team should include a surgeon, a physician (pediatric specialist), a clinical nurse practitioner or bariatric nurse, and a behavioral therapist/mental health provider (eg, psychologist, social worker, or psychiatrist).[25] Specialists in adolescent medicine and cardiology should also be included on the team.[10]

Adolescent patients require the same preoperative evaluations as adult patients (see Chapter 2). Adolescents will undergo a complete medical, including laboratory studies, psychological, social, and nutritional evaluation to determine candidacy. Cardiology, pulmonary, and gastrointestinal evaluations will be completed, as necessary. In 2018, the American Society for Metabolic and Bariatric Surgery (ASMBS) updated the selection criteria for adolescents seeking to undergo MBS. See Box 6.1 on page 132 for a complete listing of criteria.

Selection Guidelines for Adolescent Metabolic and Bariatric Surgery

Box 6.1 reviews criteria to evaluate adolescent candidates considering MBS.[18-21]

BOX 6.1 Patient Selection Criteria for Adolescent Candidates for Metabolic and Bariatric Surgery[17-19,20,25]

Health status

BMI 35 or greater or 120% of the 95th percentile plus major comorbidity (type 2 diabetes, obstructive sleep apnea, apnea-hypopnea index greater than 5, idiopathic intracranial hypertension, Blount disease, slipped capital femoral epiphysis, gastroesophogeal reflux disease, hypertension , nonalcoholic steatohepatitis) or

BMI 40 or higher or 140% of the 95th percentile (whichever is lower)

Other selection criteria

Demonstrated commitment of patient to comprehensive medical and psychological evaluations before and after metabolic and bariatric surgery (MBS)

Capability and willingness of patient to adhere to postoperative nutrition guidelines

Capacity of patient to make own decisions

Supportive family environment

Agreement to avoid becoming pregnant for at least 18 months postoperatively

Parent's and adolescent's informed consent to surgery

Developmental delay, autism spectrum, or syndromic obesity should not be a contraindication to MBS. Each patient and caregiver team will need to be assessed for ability to make dietary and lifestyle changes required and considered on a case-by-case basis

Contraindications

Current lactation or planned pregnancy within 18 months of procedure

Active substance abuse

Inadequate social/family support

Medically correctable causes of obesity

Unwillingness or inability to fully comprehend the surgical procedure and its consequences, such as lifelong medical surveillance

Medical, psychiatric, or cognitive condition affecting patient's ability to adhere to the postoperative diet or medical regimens

Evaluating Family Support

A review of the family, family support, and home environment should be part of the assessment. As adolescents' executive function is not fully developed, assessment of family support and relationships is key, as those with strong family support have improved outcomes.[26] However, the definition of *family* differs for the adolescent patient. It focuses on the location where significant time is routinely spent to identify where food/meals are purchased and available for consumption.

Preoperative Nutrition Assessment

Preoperative nutrition assessment for adolescents is similar to nutrition assessment for adults (see Chapter 2 Evaluation and Nutrition Care of Preoperative Patients). The 2015 position statement by ASMBS on metabolic bone changes after MBS states there is no need to obtain a dual-energy x-ray absorptiometry (DEXA) scan on all adolescents with severe obesity prior to MBS.[27] In the 2020 update to this paper, ASMBS recommends routine preoperative screening for the presence of vitamin D deficiency and hyperparathyroidism with treatment initiation for all patients.[28]

Additional nutritional factors to consider specific to adolescent needs include energy requirements specific to height, sex, and age and hours of screen time (eg, TV, computer, and video games, per day). Frequency of meal skipping and location of meals consumed should also be assessed. Social factors including weight-based teasing and social exclusion are likely to contribute to the desire to eat alone or to skip meals. Because adolescents with severe obesity report severe impairments in health and weight-related quality of life,[3] it is important to use motivational interviewing techniques to assist with behavior change while offering empathy and support (see Appendix H on use of education and counseling techniques).

Preoperative Education

There is a lack of evidence regarding the length and frequency of preoperative visits needed by adolescent MBS candidates.[26] Similar to adults, insurance approval for adolescent MBS candidates may require 3 to 6 months of medically supervised visits before surgery as well as psychological evaluation to demonstrate assent and a supportive environment.[29] During this time, the patient's commitment, motivation, expectations, and understanding of MBS goals are evaluated. This period also gives the adolescent an opportunity to build the knowledge and confidence needed to determine if they will choose to fully assent for MBS. Box 6.2 includes nutrition interventions for the adolescent patient during the preoperative time.

BOX 6.2 Preoperative Nutrition Interventions for Adolescent Patients (3 to 6 Months Before Metabolic and Bariatric Surgery)

Correct any identified preoperative nutritional deficiencies via supplementation and nutrition counseling.

Review food choices, meal planning, food portions, and label reading.

Review dietary modifications specific to the proposed procedure.

At each visit, work with the patient to set measurable and attainable nutrition goals that reinforce desired postoperative eating patterns in school, home-based, or work settings.

Teach mindful eating skills and how to identify hunger/fullness.

Implement a tracking system of daily intake (eg, handwritten food logs, emailing/texting daily food intake, or web or smartphone applications).

Have patient taste-test protein drinks and choose products or flavors for preoperative and postoperative consumption.

Educate the patient and family about the postoperative diet.

Recent reviews have recommended that the preoperative period should be used to build evidence-based skills that are connected to total weight loss and weight regain following MBS. In youth, these include the skills to select food choices that will assist with meeting postoperative nutrient needs, to manage eating behaviors (eg, loss of control, eating with mindfulness), to increase physical activity practices including both aerobic and strength-based activities, and to demonstrate consistent use of nutrition supplementation. As family support is key for an adolescent's postoperative success, the preoperative period gives families time to build strong support systems.[26] Although preoperative visits are frequently done with both the youth and parent/guardian together, giving youth time alone with providers affords them opportunity to speak candidly about MBS and other risk-taking behaviors. Preoperative education should be individualized to the patient's learning style (eg, auditory vs visual learning style) and presented in written, visual, or electronic formats.[18,19]

Preoperative Weight Loss

In 2016, the ASMBS updated its position on preoperative weight loss. The position stated that, "insurance-mandated preoperative weight loss is not supported by medical evidence and thus has not been shown to be effective for preoperative weight loss before MBS or to provide any benefit for bariatric outcomes."[30] Like adults, there is no evidence to support preoperative weight loss for adolescents seeking MBS.[26]

Use of a 2-week preoperative reduced calorie, reduced carbohydrate diet for the purpose of reducing liver size ahead of MBS is done with adolescents much like adults. The use of meal replacement products (eg, meal replacement shakes/bars or frozen, calorie managed meals) for all or a portion of meals is common. See Box 6.3 on page 136 for a sample preoperative diet.

Inpatient Nutrition

The average length of stay (LOS) for adolescents undergoing MBS is 2 days.[31,32] However, as more recent data sets are reviewed, published median LOS for those undergoing SG is down trending to 1.7 days.[32] Much like adults, an increasing percentage of adolescents undergoing SG are spending 0 to 1 days in the hospital following surgery.[31] A unique feature of pediatric hospitals is the role of the child-life specialist, who

BOX 6.3 Sample Preoperative Reduced Calorie and Reduced Carbohydrate Diet for Adolescent Metabolic and Bariatric Surgery Patients

Energy intake:	1,000 to 1,200 kcal/d; less than 50 g carbohydrate per day
Meals 1, 2, and 3:	Portioned, higher protein meal replacement product (eg, protein shake or protein bar) and supplemented with nonstarchy vegetables if desired
Meal 4:	Solid food meal with less than 30 g carbohydrate, supplemented with nonstarchy vegetables
Protein goal:	60 g/d or 1.0 g/kg ideal body weight (based on weight associated with body mass index of 25 for age or gender)
Fluid goal:	48 to 64 oz or more (water and sugar-free, noncarbonated, caffeine-free fluids)

may assist adolescents develop coping strategies in the immediate postoperative stage, especially for those who have increased anxiety or who experience postoperative concerns.

Postoperative dietary advancement protocols for teens are similar to adults. Teens begin their postsurgical nutrition typically on the day of surgery with a sugar-free clear liquid diet (see Appendix B about the progression of diet stages). Box 6.4 outlines the role of the RDN during the adolescent patient's hospital stay.

Postoperative Care

Postsurgical follow-up involves a multidisciplinary team with clinical expertise working with adolescents. Closer postoperative follow-up by the medical team (eg, increased visit frequency[26] and telephone or text outreach between visits) and enhanced support systems at home may contribute to adolescent patient outcomes that match or exceed adult outcomes.[32] One key objective of care is encouraging patients to be

BOX 6.4 Role of the Registered Dietitian Nutritionist in Inpatient Care of the Adolescent Metabolic and Bariatric Surgery Patient

Ensure that the adolescent and family understand the progression of the diet used during and immediately after the hospital stay.

Ensure that self-monitoring of fluid intake has begun.

Provide ample opportunity for the family to ask questions.

Confirm that the family has necessary products and equipment to advance dietary stages after discharge.

Remind patients to expand their daily postdischarge tracking to include vitamin and mineral supplementation, fluid intake, full liquid beverages consumed, and physical activity.

Provide family with tracking forms.

BOX 6.5 Suggested Follow-Up Visit Schedule for Adolescent Metabolic and Bariatric Surgery Patients

First year after surgery:

- At 2 weeks, 6 weeks, 3 months, 6 months, 9 months, 1 year
- Additional follow-up visits may be scheduled at any time, depending on the individual patient's adjustment to the diet and exercise regimen and medical needs

Second year after surgery: at 18 months and 24 months

Third year after surgery and for life: annually

appropriately independent with their postoperative care. Box 6.5 reviews postoperative visits for adolescents undergoing MBS.

The multidisciplinary team should assist the adolescent and family with the eventual transition to a facility that treats adult MBS patients or their primary care physician (PCP). If the adolescent chooses to have follow-up visits through the PCP, the RDN or advanced practice registered nurses should provide the family and the PCP with a list of nutrition supplement recommendations and a laboratory follow-up schedule.

Ongoing access to counseling from a behavioral psychologist/therapist or social worker throughout the postoperative stage can be key for adolescents making their way through changes in school, jobs, or home settings. A behavioral therapist can help ensure that the desired healthy behaviors that reinforce the anatomic and physiologic effects of MBS become habits for the patient.

Postoperative Nutrition Assessment

Postoperative nutrition monitoring and assessment is similar to that of the adult MBS patient (see Chapter 3 Nutrition Care in the Immediate Postoperative Period). Unique nutrition-related situations for adolescents undergoing MBS are presented in Box 6.6.

Laboratory tests should be obtained and assessed at the 6-, 12-, and 18-month visits and then annually for the rest of the patient's life (see Appendix D).

In adolescents, echocardiography is done 12 months after MBS if the preoperative echocardiogram was abnormal. The position statement by ASMBS on metabolic bone changes after MBS states postoperative monitoring of albumin, calcium, parathyroid hormone (PTH), and 25-hydroxyvitamin D levels is advised for bone loss monitoring.[28,33] Use of DEXA may be warranted in those who do not have stable nutritional laboratories, depending upon practitioner preference.[32]

Postoperative Nutrition Interventions

Immediate Postoperative Considerations

Hydration

The fluid intake recommendation for adolescents is the same as that for adults: a minimum of 48 to 64 oz of total fluids per day, made up of water or sugar-free noncarbonated drinks.[18] Many teens have later

BOX 6.6 Nutrition Considerations for Adolescents in the Postoperative Phase

Registered dietitian nutritionists may need to

Communicate with school food service personnel to help students get access to foods/drinks that are appropriate for each postoperative stage.

Provide employers with documentation that supports the need for established meal breaks and the ability to keep water at workstations (if appropriate).

Communicate with college/university food services to advocate for reduced meal plan options.

Communicate with athletic coaches about selection of pregame and postgame meals and protein shakes.

Help adolescents develop specific plans to use when eating out with friends in social situations or away from school at competitive events (eg, band competitions, academic events, athletic events).

Advocate with school medical providers or nurses to provide adolescents with a private place to eat meals in the immediate postoperative phase for those adolescents who desire to keep their metabolic and bariatric surgery a private matter.

Monitor weight loss velocity, assess for nutrition etiologies, and intervene with nutritional plans as needed.

day sleep-wake patterns, which may make it difficult for parents or caregivers to keep up with how much fluid the teen is drinking in the immediate postoperative period, especially if they drink the majority of their fluids later in the evening. Setting up a system, such as using a tracking app or sheet or placing a set number of water bottles onto the countertop for teens to drink, can be very helpful for parents and teens to monitor hydration in the first weeks after surgery. Once teens return to school, they will need to carry a water bottle with them throughout the day. Students may need written permission from medical providers to carry a water bottle with them and to have access to water throughout the school day.

Diet Progression

As discussed in Chapter 3, advancement of the postoperative diet varies slightly depending on the type of MBS procedure (see also Appendix B). Adolescent patients, like adult patients, will vary on their progression through the various diet phases. Using a patient-centered approach will allow the dietitian to move the patient along at a pace that is comfortable for the patient yet reinforces the anatomic and physiologic effects of MBS. For some adolescents, this may mean breaking up postoperative dietary progressions into substages that can accommodate school schedules as well as after schoolwork or athletic schedules.

Protein Intake

To maintain lean body mass, promote healing, and minimize hair loss, many MBS programs recommend a dietary intake range of 60 to 80 g protein per day (1.0 g/kg ideal body weight, based on weight associated with a BMI of 25 for age and gender) after MBS.[18,34,35] The adolescent patient should aim to eat 15 to 20 g protein from high-bioavailability protein sources at each of three to five meals per day, based upon pouch volume tolerance (see Chapter 3 for sample meal ideas during diet stages). One small study ($n = 11$) assessed changes in body composition of adolescents with severe obesity undergoing RYGB surgery. Fat-free mass (FFM) declined primarily in the first 6 weeks after surgery, with limited, nonsignificant changes noted in FFM through the 12-month assessment point. Total FFM decreased by −12% + or −5% of initial FFM.[36]

Vitamin and Mineral Supplementation

Following MBS, adolescent patients need lifelong daily vitamin and mineral supplementation similar to adult needs. See Appendix C for a complete list of vitamin/mineral recommendations.

Micronutrients of concern in the postoperative phase for adolescents include risk for deficiencies of iron, vitamin B12, vitamin D, and thiamine (vitamin B1). In a study that focused on adherence to use of micronutrient supplementation in adolescents 5 years after RYGB, iron deficiency anemia continued to have a high prevalence.[37] Similar concerns with iron deficiency were also found in adolescents 2 years after SG, possibly due to decreased hydrochloric acid production essential for iron absorption after gastric resection, along with reduced intake of iron-rich food, such as red meat. Iron deficiency anemia warrants close postoperative monitoring (especially for those assigned female at birth) for anemia. In adolescents, reduced bone mass was noted 2 years after MBS; however, it remained appropriate for age and new body weight.[38] Elevated parathyhroid levels were found in the adolescents who underwent RYGB 5 years prior, regardless of vitamin supplement adherence.[37] In 2-year postoperative SG adolescents, postoperative vitamin D deficiency and secondary hyperparathyroidism were also a concern.[37] The authors recommend ongoing assessment of the optimal vitamin D and calcium supplementation doses needed to preserve bone health.[38]

Adherence to use of micronutrient supplementation is not well documented in adolescents. In one study of adolescents who underwent RYGB 5 years prior, data indicated a generally higher and better maintained micronutrient status in participants who adhered to dietary supplementation. The findings from this study were in line with other studies of adolescents with chronic illness, reporting adherence to long-term chronic disease regimens averaging 50%.[37] This is in contrast to a second study that found lower adherence rates for use of nutritional supplements by teens undergoing MBS. An electronic monitoring cap was placed onto multivitamin bottles and tracked the dates and times the bottles were opened and closed by adolescents both prior to and following weight loss surgery. Declining adherence was noted over the first 6 postoperative months, finding mean adherence for the entire 6-month period was approximately 30%. Initially following surgery, forgetting to take vitamins was the primary barrier that then shifted to difficulty swallowing vitamins.[39]

The RDN should help to inform the adolescent about multiple supplement options (eg, chewable, tablet, liquid) and work with the adolescent to help find a supplement that they are willing to take. Many teens are interested in supplements that they can conveniently carry on the go like individually wrapped multivitamin or calcium soft chews or multivitamin stick packs. The RDN should also help patients devise strategies to optimize adherence to multivitamin therapy, which may be challenging for adolescents. Use of cell phone reminders and alarms or specific apps for medication use may enhance supplement use in adolescents.[39]

Longer-Term Considerations

Environmental Influences

Nutrition intervention after MBS requires focused attention on how the adolescent patient's environment affects the patient's behaviors. The RDN should help patients identify environmental triggers to unhealthy eating and nonphysical hunger and work with them to manage these triggers at postoperative visits. Education regarding how surgery affects hunger and satiety levels (see Chapter 1) is crucial, and patients should receive ongoing nutrition counseling to manage potential setbacks. See Chapter 3 for examples of relevant nutrition interventions.

Many environmental factors that may affect the nutrition intervention should be considered as the patient enters adulthood. For example, patients may change their living arrangements when they attend college or technical school, start a job, or get married. At such times, patients may need assistance in determining how the changes affect their eating regimen (eg, goals, portion sizes, and fluid choices) and behaviors.

Energetic Adaptations

Four studies evaluated energetic and metabolic adaptations in adolescents undergoing MBS.[36,40-42] Of the three studies reporting pre- and post-MBS resting energy expenditure (REE) data, all reported absolute REE[40,42] or BMR[36] decreased over the first year following MBS. However, when controlling for total body weight (TBW), Rickard and colleagues[43] reported an increase in REE/TBW in post-MBS adolescents. Brehm and colleagues[41] also reported no difference in REE/TBW or REE controlled for fat-free mass in post-MBS adolescents compared with weight-stable, matched controls who did not undergo MBS. In the study by Rickard and colleagues,[42] changes in REE/TBW for post-MBS patients strongly correlated with percent total weight loss at 1 year. Data from Butte and colleagues[36] differed, finding a decrease in total daily energy expenditure per kilogram FFM in post-RYGB patients at 2 months and persisting through 1 year after surgery. Metabolic adaptation studies in adults undergoing MBS also show mixed results.

Data regarding calorie intake following MBS in adolescents is limited. Brehm and colleagues[41] reported weight-stable, post-SG patients reported lower daily caloric intake compared with their matched weight-stable, nonsurgical controls, despite little difference in measured REE values. Complex interactions and changes to endocrine adaptations following MBS may contribute to energetic adaptations occurring after MBS. Further long-term study of the impact of MBS on REE and total daily energy expenditure is needed in youth undergoing MBS to understand if these adaptations are transient or will persist, as research on the impact of MBS on resting metabolic rate (RMR) in adults is inconsistent.[36]

As discussed in Chapter 4, clinicians typically use predictive equations or indirect calorimetry to assess a patient's RMR and energy requirements. The Mifflin-St. Jeor (for BMI higher than 30) is typically used in adolescents with severe obesity.[43] Although the Mifflin-St. Jeor was validated in youth with severe obesity,[43] at the individual level underestimation or overestimation of energy needs can challenge its clinical usefulness.[42] Indirect calorimetry can provide a more accurate RMR value under proper testing conditions. Because of these limitations, RDNs should exercise caution when using predictive equations or indirect calorimetry in this patient population, as results may not be accurate.

Therefore, instead of setting calorie limits, the RDN should counsel adolescent patients whose weight has stabilized and appetite signals have returned to regulate their energy intake by paying attention to their hunger and satiety and practicing mindful eating.[42,44] Including mindful eating strategies along with nutrition guidelines used for weight maintenance can help to foster a concomitant healthy relationship with food.

Alcohol Use

In adults undergoing MBS, there is strong evidence to show increased risk of developing problems with alcohol use in the postoperative phase, ranging from increased alcohol use to alcohol use disorder.[45] MBS appears to increase the risk of alcohol misuse postoperatively. Only one study has evaluated alcohol use risk in adolescents undergoing MBS compared with a nonsurgical control group. The majority of participants in the study were nondrinkers. However, for the surgical group only, alcohol use prevalence changed significantly with increasing age and as a function of decreasing BMI. As teens age, they will have greater opportunities to try alcohol for the first time. Practitioners should screen routinely for alcohol use behavior in the preoperative and postoperative phases. Education that promotes abstinence and that discusses harm reduction related to drinking is crucial for teens entering into young adult years.[46]

Loss of Control Eating

Loss of control (LOC) eating is defined as a sense that one cannot control what or how much one is eating.[47] LOC eating in the postoperative period is linked with poorer weight outcomes in adults who underwent MBS. One study reviewed LOC eating in adolescents undergoing MBS, and similar findings were reported for teens as adults. Reported LOC eating at the 1-, 2-, and 3-year follow-up visit was predictive of greater subsequent weight regain in teens undergoing MBS. Specifically, researchers found that LOC eating that matches grazing, eating small amounts of food continuously in an unplanned matter, was more strongly linked with weight regain.[49] Evaluating for LOC eating in annual follow-up visits is warranted when meeting with teens.

Reproductive and Sexual Health Care

Adolescent MBS programs should include counseling and recommendations regarding reproductive health concerns and sexual health outcomes as part of the preoperative and postoperative assessments. Alternatively, patients could be referred to professionals familiar with common reproductive health problems among people with severe obesity.[18]

Infertility decreases after MBS.[20] However, as discussed in Chapter 7, MBS patients should avoid planned pregnancy for 12 to 18 months after surgery.[21,49] Counseling about appropriate methods to prevent pregnancy should be provided to any young person planning to have MBS.

Adolescence is a time of evolving sexual practices. In a study of adolescents undergoing MBS, "the majority of them experienced sexual debut during the four years following surgery, which is consistent with age-normative trends." However, adolescents that have been through MBS reported more sexual risk behaviors than their nonsurgical peers.[48]

Bariatric surgical programs for teens should include ongoing counseling on teen's evolving sexual practices, including pregnancy education, sexually transmitted infections/HIV prevention, and the impact of substance use on sexual decision-making. Asking sexual orientation and gender identity questions is critically important given the health disparities in the lesbian, gay, bisexual, and transgender community.[48]

Postoperative Nutrition Diagnosis

Refer to Chapter 3 and Appendix E for examples of nutrition diagnoses relevant in the postoperative period.

Postoperative Monitoring and Evaluation

Lifelong follow-up with the multidisciplinary team and education of the PCP are crucial in maintaining the long-term outcomes of the patient. RDNs must continually monitor each patient's nutritional status and evaluate and document the outcomes of nutrition interventions. As the number of adolescent MBS procedures increases, continued research and long-term outcome data need to be collected and shared as a basis for future treatment decisions for adolescents worldwide.

References

1. Skinner AC, Rayanbakht SH, Skelton JA, Perrin EM, Armstrong SC. Prevalence of obesity and severe obesity in US Children, 1999-201. *Pediatrics*. 2018;141(3):e20173459. doi:10.1542/peds.2018-1916
2. Weiss R, Dziura J, Burgert TS, et al. Obesity and the metabolic syndrome in children and adolescents. *N Engl J Med*. 2004;350(23):2362-2374. doi:10.1056/NEJMoa031049
3. Zeller MH, Roehrig HR, Modi AC, Daniels SR, Inge TH. Health-related quality of life and depressive symptoms in adolescents with extreme obesity presenting for bariatric surgey. *Pediatrics*. 2006;117(4):1155-1161. doi:10.1542/peds.2005-1141
4. Wright N, Wales J. Assessment and management of severely obese children and adolescents. *Arch Dis Child*. 2016;101(12):1161-1167. doi:10.1136/archdischild-2015-309103
5. Kelly AS, Barlow SE, Rao G, et al. Severe obeisty in children and adolescents: identification, associated health risks and treatment approaches. A scientific statement from the American Heart Association. *Circulation*. 2013;128(15):1689-1712. doi:10.1161/CIR.0b013e3182a5cfb3

6. Lawson ML, Kirk S, Mitchell T, et al. One-year outcomes of Roux-en-Y gastric bypass for morbidly obese adolescents: a multicenter study from the Pediatric Bariatric Study Group. *J Pediatr Surg*. 2006;41(1):137-143. doi:10.1016/j.jpedsurg.2005.10.017
7. Messiah SE, Lopez-Mitnik G, Winegar D, et al. Changes in weight and co-morbidities among adolescents undergoing bariatric surgery: 1-year results from the Bariatric Outcomes Longitudinal Database. *Surg Obes Relat Dis*. 2013;9(4):503-513. doi:10.1016/j.soard.2012.03.007
8. Jen HC, Rickard DG, Shew SB, et al. Trends and outcomes of adolescent bariatric surgery in California, 2005-2007. *Pediatrics*. 2010;126(4):e746-e753. doi:10.1542/peds.2010-0412
9. De La Cruz-Muñoz N, Lopez-Mitnik G, Arheart K, Miller TL, Lipshultz SE, Messiah SE. Effectiveness of bariatric surgery in reducing weight and body mass index among Hispanic adolescents. *Obes Surg*. 2013;23(2):150-156. doi:10.1007/s11695-012-0730-0
10. Inge TH, Jenkins TM, Zeller M, et al. Baseline BMI is a strong predictor of nadir BMI after adolescent gastric bypass. *J Pediatr*. 2010;156(1):103-108. doi:10.1016/j.jpeds.2009.07.028
11. Paulus G, de Vaan LEG, Verdam FJ, BouvyND, Ambergen TA, Van Heurn LW. Bariatric surgery in morbidly obese adolescents: a systematic review and meta-analysis. *Obes Surg*. 2015;25(5):860-878. doi:10.1007/s11695-015-1581-2
12. Inge TH, Coley RY, Bazzano LA, et al. Comparative effectivenss of bariatric procedures among adolescents: the PCORnet bariatric study. *Surg Obes Relat Dis*. 2018;14(9):1374-1386. doi:10.1016/j.soard.2018.04.002
13. Michlsky MP, Inge TH, Jenkins TM, et al. Cardiovascular risk factors after adolescent bariatric surgery. *Pediatrics*. 2018;141(2):e20172485. doi:10.1542/peds.2017-2485
14. Armstrong SC, Gooling CG, Michalsky MP, et al.; AAP Section on Obesity, Section on Surgery. Pediatric, metabolic and bariatric surgery: evidence, barriers, and best practices. *Pediatrics*. 2019;144(6):e20193223. doi:10.1542/peds.2019-3223
15. Varela JE, Hinojosa MW, Nguyen NT. Perioperative outcomes of bariatric surgery in adolescents compared with adults at academic medical centers. *Surg Obes Relat Dis*. 2007;3(5):537-542. doi:10.1016/j.soard.2007.07.002
16. Altieri M, Pryor A, Bates A, Docimo S, Talamini M, Spaniolas K. Bariatric procedures in adolescents are safe in accredited centers. *Surg Obes Relat Dis*. 2018;14(9):1368-1372. doi:10.1016/j.soard.2018.04.004
17. Aikenhead A, Lobstein T, Knai C. Review of current guidelines on adolescent bariatric surgery. *Clin Obes*. 2011;1(1):3-11. doi:10.1111/j.1758-8111.2010.00002.x

18. Fullmer M, Abrams S, Hrovat K, et al. Nutritional strategy for the adolescent patient undergoing bariatric surgery: report of a working group of the Nutrition Committee of NASPGHAN/NACHRI [published correction appears in *J Pediatr Gastroenterol Nutr.* 2012 Apr; 54(4):571]. *J Pediatr Gastroenterol Nutr.* 2012;54(1):125-135. doi:10.1097/MPG.0b013e318231db79

19. Inge TH, Krebs NF, Garcia VF, et al. Bariatric surgery for severely overweight adolescents: concerns and recommendations. *Pediatrics.* 2004;114(1):217-223. doi:10.1542/peds.114.1.217

20. Pratt J, Lenders C, Dionne E, et al. Best practice updates for pediatric/adolescent weight loss surgery. *Obesity (Silver Spring).* 2009;17(5):901-910. doi:10.1038/oby.2008.577

21. Pratt JSA, Browne A, Browne NT, et al. ASMBS pediatric metabolic and bariatric surgery guidelines, 2018. *Surg Obes Relat Dis.* 2018;14(7):882-901. doi:10.1016/j.soard.2018.03.019

22. Lennerz BS, Wabitsch M, Lippert H, et al. Bariatric surgery in adolescents and young adults: safety and effectiveness in a cohort of 345 patients. *Int J Obes. (Lond).* 2014;38(3):334-340. doi:10.1038/ijo.2013.182

23. Inge TH, Zeller MH, Jenkis TM, et al. Perioperative outcomes of adolescents undergoing bariatric surgery: the Teen-Longitudinal Assessment of Bariatric Surgery (Teen-LABS) study. *JAMA Pediatr.* 2014;168(1):47-53. doi:10.1001/jamapediatrics.2013.4296

24. Michalsky M, Kramer RE, Fullmer MA, et al. Developing criteria for pediatric/adolescent bariatric surgery programs. *Pediatrics.* 2011;128 suppl 2:S65-S70. doi:10.1542/peds.2011-0480F

25. Standards manual. MBSAQIP standards—effective October 2019. Metabolic and Bariatric Surgery Accreditation and Quality Improvement Program. Accessed September 13, 2019. www.facs.org/quality-programs/mbsaqip/standards

26. Moore JM, Haemer MA, Fox CK. Lifestyle and pharmacologic management before and after bariatric surgery. *Semin Pediatr Surg.* 2020;29(1):150889. doi:10.1016/j.sempedsurg.2020.150889

27. Kim JJ, Rogers AM, Ballem N, Schirmer B; American Society Metabolic and Bariatric Surgery Clinical Issues Committee. American Society for Metabolic and Bariatric Surgery Clinical Issues Committee, position statement. Metabolic bone changes after bariatric surgery. *Surg Obes Relat Dis.* 2015;11(2):406-411.

28. Kim J, Nimeri A, Khogani Z, ElCjhaar M, Lima AG, Vosburg PW; American Society for Metabolic and Bariatric Surgery (ASMBS) Clinical Issues Committee. Metabolic bone changes after bariatric surgery: 2020 Update, American Society for Metabolic and Bariatric Surgery Clinical Issues Committee position statement. *Surg Obes Relat Dis.* 2021;17(1):1-8. doi:10.1016/j.soard.2020.09.031

29. Bariatric surgery. May 2020. Accessed June 15, 2020. www.uhcprovider.com/content/dam/provider/docs/public/policies/comm-medical-drug/bariatric-surgery.pdf
30. ASMBS updates position statement on insurance mandates preoperative weight loss requirements. *Surg Obes Relat Dis.* 2016;12(5):955-959. doi:10.1016/j.soard.2016.04.019
31. Kyler KE, Bettenhausen JL, Hall M, Fraser JD, Sweeney B. Trends in volume and utilization outcomes in adolescent metabolic and bariatric surgery at children's hospitals. *J Adolesc Health.* 2019;65(3):331-336. doi:10.1016/j.jadohealth.2019.02.021
32. El Chaar M, King K, Al-Mardini A, Galvez A, Claros L, Stoltzfus J. Thirty-day outcomes of bariatric surgery in adolescents a first-look at the MBSAQIP database. *Obes Surg.* 2021;31:194-199. doi:10.1007/s11695-020.040866-w
33. Kushner RF, Cummings S, Herron DM. Bariatric surgery: postoperative nutritional management. In: Jones D, ed. *UpToDate*. UpToDate; 2020. Accessed June 14, 2020. www.uptodate.com/contents/bariatric-surgery-postoperative-nutritional-management?search=bariatric-surgery-&source=search_result&selectedTitle=1~150&usage_type=default&display_rank=1
34. Mechanick JI, Kushner RF, Sugerman HJ, et al. American Association of Clinical Endocrinologists, the Obesity Society, and American Society for Metabolic & Bariatric Surgery Medical Guidelines for Clinical Practice for the perioperative nutritional, metabolic, and nonsurgical support of the bariatric surgery patient [published correction appears in *Surg Obes Relat Dis.* 2010 Jan-Feb;6(1):112]. *Surg Obes Relat Dis.* 2008;4(5 suppl):S109-S184. doi:10.1016/j.soard.2008.08.009
35. Allied Health Sciences Section Ad Hoc Nutrition Committee; Aills L, Blankenship J, Buffington C, Furtado M, Parrott J. ASMBS allied health nutritional guidelines for the surgical weight loss patient. *Surg Obes Relat Dis.* 2008;4(5 suppl):S73-S108. doi:10.1016/j.soard.2008.03.002
36. Butte NF, Brandt ML, Wong WW, et al. Energetic adaptations persist after bariatric surgery in severely obese adolescents. *Obesity (Silver Spring).* 2015;23(3):591-601. doi:10.1002/oby.20994
37. Henfridsson P, Laurenius A, Wallengren O, et al. Micronutrient intake and biochemistry in adolescents adherent or nonadherent to supplements 5 years after Roux-en-Y gastric bypass surgery. *Surg Obes Relat Dis.* 2019;15(9):1494-1502. doi:10.1016/j.soard.2019.06.012
38. Elhag, W, El Ansari W, Abdulrazzaq S, et al. Evolution of 29 anthropometric, nutritional and cardiometabolic parameters among morbidly obese adolescents 2 years post sleeve gastrectomy. *Obes Surg.* 2018;28(2):474-482. doi:10.1007/s11695-017-2868-2
39. Modi AC, Zeller MH, Xanthakos SA, Jenkins TM, Inge TH. Adherence to vitamin supplementation following adolescent bariatric surgery. *Obesity (Silver Spring).* 2013;21(3):E190-E195. doi:10.1002/oby.20031

40. Chu L, Steinberg A, Mehta M, et al. Resting energy expenditure and metabolic adaptation in adolescents at 12 Months after bariatric surgery. *J Clin Endocrinol Metab*. 2019;104(7):2648-2656. doi:10.1210/jc.2018-02244

41. Brehm B, Summer S, Jenkins T, D'Alessio D, Inge T. Thermic effect of food and resting energy expenditure after sleeve gastrectomy for weight loss in adolescent females. *Surg Obes Relat Dis*. 2020;16(5):599-606. doi:10.1016/j.soard.2020.01.025

42. Rickard FA, Torre Flores LP, Malhotra S, et al. Comparison of measured and estimated resting energy expenditure in adolescents and young adults with severe obesity before and 1 Year after sleeve gastrectomy. *Front Pediatr*. 2019;7:37. doi:10.3389/fped.2019.00037

43. Steinberg A, Manlhiot C, Cordeiro K, et al. Determining the accuracy of predictive energy expenditure (PREE) equations in severely obese adolescents. *Clin Nutr*. 2017;36(4):1158-1164. doi:10.1016/j.clnu.2016.08.006

44. van Hout GC, Verschure SK, van Heck GL. Psychosocial predictors of success following bariatric surgery. *Obes Surg*. 2005;15(4):552-560. doi:10.1381/0960892053723484

45. Ivezaj V, Benoit SC, Davis J, et al. Changes in alcohol use after metabolic and bariatric surgery: predictors and mechanisms. *Curr Psychiatry Rep*. 2019;21(9):85. doi:10.1007/s/1920-019-1070-8

46. Zeller MH, Washington GA, Mitchell JE, et al. Alcohol use risk in adolescents 2 years after bariatric surgery. *Surg Obes Relat Dis*. 2017;13(1):85-94. doi:10.1016/j.soard.2016.05.019

47. Goldschmidt AB, Khoury J, Jenkins TM, et al. Adolescent loss-of-control eating and weight loss maintenance after bariatric surgery. *Pediatrics*. 2018;141:1(1):e20171659. doi:10.1542/peds.2017-1659

48. Zeller MH, Brown JL, Reiter-Purtill J, et al. Sexual behaviors, risks, and sexual health outcomes for adolescent females following bariatric surgery. *Surg Obes Relat Dis*. 2019;15(6):969-978. doi:10.1016/j.soard.2019.03.001

49. Wagner CL, Greer FR. American Academy of Pediatrics section on breastfeeding; American Academy of Pediatrics committee on nutrition. Prevention of rickets and vitamin D deficiency in infants, children, and adolescents [published correction appears in *Pediatrics*. 2009 Jan;123(1):197]. *Pediatrics*. 2008;122(5):1142-1152. doi:10.1542/peds.2008-1862

CHAPTER 7

Special Considerations After Metabolic and Bariatric Surgery

Introduction

This chapter addresses the following special considerations related to metabolic and bariatric surgery (MBS) that are not covered in detail elsewhere in this pocket guide:

- postbariatric hypoglycemia
- type 1 diabetes mellitus
- renal disease and transplantation
- pregnancy

Postbariatric Hypoglycemia

Postbariatric hypoglycemia (PBH) is also referred to as postprandial hyperinsulinemic hypoglycemia or reactive hypoglycemia. It may also be referred to as "late dumping syndrome," which is different from "dumping syndrome." There is no agreed-upon diagnostic criteria for PBH since presentation can be nonspecific.[1] However, criteria typically include presentation of Whipple's triad for hypoglycemia within 1 to 3 hours of consuming a meal high in carbohydrate content.[1,2] The triad includes the following:

- symptomatic hypoglycemia
- perspiration
- palpitations
- hunger
- weakness
- confusion
- tremor
- syncope
- low blood glucose, typically below 50 to 60 mg/dL[1]
- resolution of symptoms after administration of glucose

It is important to note that glucose in the fasting state is normal in patients who experience PBH.[3]

Etiology

Patients most commonly experience PBH 12 to 24 months or later after MBS. PBH has been diagnosed up to 4 years postoperatively.[1,4,5] Refer to Box 7.1 for a list of possible MBS-related etiologies of PBH.[3,6]

PBH is underreported, making it difficult to determine the prevalence of PBH after MBS. However, the majority of patients who undergo MBS will not experience PBH. Data from the Bariatric Outcomes Longitudinal Database (BOLD) study suggest that the incidence of self-reported hypoglycemia after RYGB is 0.1%. PBH occurs in both Roux-en-Y gastric bypass (RYGB) patients and sleeve gastrectomy (SG) patients. Severe hypoglycemic events are more likely to occur in RYGB patients vs SG patients. PBH is not a complication of adjustable gastric band (AGB) or gastric balloons.[1]

BOX 7.1 Possible Etiologies of Postbariatric Hypoglycemia[3,6]

Alterations in glucose regulatory mechanisms

β cell hyperfunction

Underlying familial hyperinsulinism syndrome (unmasked by weight loss)

Increased insulin sensitivity secondary to weight loss

Increased β cell mass that developed during obesity and did not regress postoperatively

Excess secretion of glucagon-like peptide 1

Increased delivery of nutrients to the intestines after Roux-en-Y gastric bypass or sleeve gastrectomy

Nutrition Assessment

To assess patients for PBH, the registered dietitian nutritionist (RDN) should ask them to keep a record including blood glucose levels, timing of meals, food and fluids consumed, and details on when symptoms occur.

Interventions

Nutrition Intervention

Treatment for patients with post-MBS hypoglycemia parallels treatment for patients with hypoglycemia unrelated to MBS. Low-carbohydrate diets can prevent or improve symptoms of PBH.[7] Generally, consuming small, frequent meals and avoiding refined carbohydrates can help reduce the occurrence of PBH (see Box 7.2).[2,4]

Pharmacological Treatment

Patients who do not respond to dietary treatment for PBH should be referred to an endocrinologist for further evaluation. The endocrinologist and dietitian can collaborate regarding the patient's care. These

BOX 7.2 Diet for Managing or Preventing Reactive Hypoglycemia[2,4]

Control portions of carbohydrates.

Include protein and heart-healthy fats at meals and snacks.

Avoid all added sugars and refined carbohydrates in foods and beverages.

Chew food thoroughly and slowly.

Consume a meal or snack every 3 to 4 hours.

Do not drink large amounts of fluid with or immediately following a meal.

Maintain blood glucose levels during exercise.

patients may need medications in addition to dietary interventions (see Box 7.3 on page 154).[1,4]

Surgical Treatment

Severe cases of PBH due to hyperplasia of the β cells or nesidioblastosis have been reported in a few RYGB patients. In these cases, a partial or total pancreatic resection may be warranted.[5,9,10] Revision surgery to reverse the RYGB may be considered if the patient has exhausted all other forms of treatment and continues to experience hypoglycemic symptoms that are compromising quality of life.[1,6]

Nutrition Monitoring and Evaluation

The patient and RDN should evaluate the frequency and occurrence of symptoms of PBH. Box 7.4 on page 155 lists the steps the RDN should use in the monitoring and evaluation process.

Type 1 Diabetes

Approximately 50% of adults with type 1 diabetes have overweight or obesity.[11] Despite the rising prevalence of obesity in this cohort, there is limited data on type 1 diabetes and MBS.[12-14] In the few studies conducted, the most significant change observed has been a decrease in the

BOX 7.3 Medications Used to Manage Postbariatric Hypoglycemia[1,4,8]

Acarbose (Precose)

Route of administration	Oral
Mechanism of action	Delays the breakdown of starch into sugar
Adverse effects	Bloating, flatulence, diarrhea

Nifedipine (Procardia XL)

Route of administration	Oral
Mechanism of action	Reduces insulin secretion
Adverse effects	Nausea, hypotension, constipation

Diazoxide (Proglycem)

Route of administration	Oral
Mechanism of action	Reduces insulin secretion
Adverse effects	Hypotension, nausea, vomiting

Glucagon-like peptide 1 analogs

Route of administration	Injectable
Mechanism of action	Block the action of glucagon-like peptide 1, suppress postprandial insulin secretion
Adverse effects	Nausea, vomiting, diarrhea, headache, weakness, dizziness

Ocreotide (Sandostatin)

Route of administration	Injectable
Mechanism of action	Delays gastric emptying; slows transit through the bowel; inhibits insulin secretion, postprandial vasodilation, and the release of gastrointestinal hormones
Adverse effects	Gallstone formation, pain at injection site, steatorrhea

BOX 7.4 Monitoring and Evaluation for Postbariatric Hypoglycemia

Nutrition self-monitoring at agreed-upon rate
Initiate patient self-monitoring of blood glucose. The patient tracks blood glucose levels before and after meals via a glucometer.

Nutrition self-monitoring at agreed-upon rate
If a continuous glucose monitoring device is available, the patient should use it with a glucometer.

Total carbohydrate estimated intake in 24 hours
Initiate tracking of food intake and symptoms. This record allows the registered dietitian nutritionist to analyze intake to determine patterns between food consumed and low blood glucose or symptoms of reactive hypoglycemia.

total daily insulin dose after MBS (particularly RYGB). This decrease is directly related to weight loss and increased insulin sensitivity. The benefits of using less insulin include the decrease of body fat accumulation and cost savings for the patient. Some—but not all—studies show improved glycemic control after surgery.[14-16] In addition, research has shown an improvement in cardiovascular disease risk factors.[14,17] Further research on type 1 diabetes and MBS is needed.

Nutrition Assessment

The RDN must work closely with the patient's endocrinologist to properly assess and titrate the insulin dose(s) immediately after MBS. Box 7.5 on page 156 to 157 includes factors to consider when assessing glucose control in patients with type 1 diabetes.[18]

Nutrition Diagnosis

Nutrition diagnoses for MBS patients with type 1 diabetes are typically based on data from the patient's food recall, food record, or laboratory values. Box 7.6 on page 157 lists nutrition diagnoses often used with patients with type 1 diabetes.[13]

BOX 7.5 Factors to Consider in the Nutrition Assessment of Patients With Type 1 Diabetes[18,19]

Need for sliding-scale vs fixed insulin doses

Some patients are on a sliding scale according to the premeal blood glucose reading. The higher the blood glucose, the more insulin is needed.

For fixed insulin doses, the amount of carbohydrates consumed revolves around the amount of insulin given. Therefore, if fewer carbohydrates are consumed than recommended for that insulin dose, there is a risk for hypoglycemia.

Total carbohydrate intake and carbohydrate-to-insulin ratio

As carbohydrate intake decreases, less insulin is required.

In addition, as body weight decreases, the total daily insulin dose decreases as well; calculate new total daily doses and new carbohydrate-to-insulin ratios during weight loss.

Calculating total daily insulin dose: $\frac{\textit{Actual weight in lb}}{4}$

Calculating carbohydrate-to-insulin ratio ("500 Rule"): $\frac{500}{\textit{total daily insulin dose}}$

Calculating correction factor: $\frac{1{,}800}{\text{total daily insulin dose}}$

Timing of insulin injection

Most patients inject rapid-acting insulin premeal.

However, considering the risk of vomiting and food intolerances after metabolic and bariatric surgery (MBS), injecting insulin at the completion of the meal may be advised because this may help reduce the risk of hypoglycemia.

Risks of hypoglycemia

For most patients, carbohydrate intake dramatically decreases after MBS. If insulin is not adjusted based on the new carbohydrate intake, there is a risk for hypoglycemia.

Exercise and physical activity

Activity can increase the risk for hypoglycemia. Educate patients on how activity affects their blood glucose.

Preworkout and postworkout blood glucose readings are useful.

BOX 7.5 Factors to Consider in the Nutrition Assessment of Patients With Type 1 Diabetes[18,19] (cont.)

Diabetic ketoacidosis

Symptoms include nausea, vomiting, hyperglycemia, and high ketones. The incidence of diabetic ketoacidosis may be up to one in four. It is typically a result of poor oral intake, poor perioperative insulin adjustment, dehydration, or infection.

Euglycemic ketoacidosis is rare but can be caused by reduced carbohydrate intake in type 1 diabetes patients post–MBS. Symptoms occur in the setting of normal blood glucose levels. Serum ketones and blood gas analysis should be performed to confirm diagnosis.

BOX 7.6 Selected Nutrition Diagnoses for Patients With Type 1 Diabetes[20]

Inconsistent carbohydrate intake

Carbohydrate intake is not evenly distributed throughout meals and snacks

Excessive carbohydrate intake

Daily carbohydrate intake exceeds estimated needs, which is 50% of total calorie intake

Altered nutrition-related laboratory values

Blood work reveals blood glucose and hemoglobin A1c are above the normal range

Nutrition Intervention, Monitoring, and Evaluation

Box 7.7 on page 158 lists possible nutrition interventions for the patient with type 1 diabetes before and after MBS. Refer to Boxes 7.8 and 7.9 on page 159 for information about preventing and treating hypoglycemia in patients with type 1 diabetes.[18]

BOX 7.7 Preoperative and Postoperative Nutrition Interventions for Metabolic and Bariatric Surgery Patients With Type 1 Diabetes[18]

Preoperative diet

Nutrition counseling based on self-monitoring strategy	Monitor blood glucose closely to prevent hypoglycemia while on a restricted carbohydrate diet.
Carbohydrate-modified diet	Recommend beverages with higher carbohydrate content, such as protein shakes, milk, or soy milk.

Postoperative diet[a]

Specific foods/beverages or groups	Recommend calorie-free, sugar-free clear liquids (clear liquid).
Consistent carbohydrate diet	Recommend protein shakes with higher carbohydrate content (full liquid).
Nutrition counseling based on self-monitoring strategy	Monitor intake of carbohydrates aiming for ~50 g carbohydrate per day, and monitor blood glucose closely (semisolid or soft foods).
Decreased carbohydrate diet	50% of total energy intake should comprise carbohydrate (regular textures).

[a] Currently, there is no research on type 1 diabetes and preoperative and postoperative diets. Metabolic and bariatric surgery patients with type 1 diabetes follow the same guidelines as all other postoperative patients, but they eventually aim for the Recommended Dietary Allowance of 130 g carbohydrate (~50% of total calories) when they make it to the final stage.

BOX 7.8 Treatment of Hypoglycemia in Type 1 Diabetes[18]

A blood glucose measurement less than 70 mg/dL is considered indicative of hypoglycemia; however, some patients experience symptoms at higher levels. It is best to treat based on the patient's symptoms.

Treatment recommendation:

- Patients should take 15 to 20 g glucose or other simple carbohydrates. Glucose tablets are preferred. These can be purchased at a pharmacy. Each glucose tablet contains 4 g glucose. Some patients, particularly Roux-en-Y gastric bypass patients, cannot tolerate glucose tablets; food/liquid sources of sugar (eg, diluted juice) are an alternative for these patients.
- Patients should recheck blood glucose 15 minutes after treatment. If blood glucose is still low, they should retreat and check blood glucose again until blood glucose more than 70 mg/dL.
- After treating hypoglycemia, patients should consume a balanced snack that contains protein and fiber to stabilize blood glucose.
- Patients should recheck blood glucose 60 minutes after the snack to confirm that the glucose level is within the normal range.

BOX 7.9 Strategies to Prevent Hypoglycemia in Patients with Type 1 Diabetes

Communication with patient's endocrinologist to adjust insulin dose accordingly as patient loses weight.

Self-monitor preprandial and postprandial blood glucose with a glucometer.

Continuously monitor glucose with a tracking device that measures glucose levels in interstitial fluids throughout the day and alert the patient of low or drastic decreases in blood glucose, as well as high glucose levels.

Check hemoglobin A1c every 3, 6, or 12 months, depending on blood glucose control.

Determine frequency of hypoglycemia and develop strategies to prevent it.

Track food and liquid intake and symptoms.

Renal Disease and Transplantation

Kidney function of some patients with renal disease improves substantially after MBS, making early intervention ideal.[21] However, once an individual reaches end-stage renal failure and dialysis, the goal is typically renal transplant. Most transplant programs and systems require patients be under a certain body mass index (BMI) in order to be listed for an organ. This has led to MBS being more commonly used as a bridge to organ transplantation for individuals who may not otherwise have been candidates.[22] MBS has been shown to increase the likelihood of transplantation and minimize posttransplant weight gain in those who eventually receive an organ.[23]

End-Stage Renal Disease

The nutritional requirements for MBS patients with end-stage renal disease ESRD (chronic kidney disease [CKD] stage 5) are challenging. Bariatric RDNs and renal dietitians should work together to assess patients and advise them on the preoperative and postoperative diet and supplementation. The renal dialysis team should collect and monitor data about fluid, protein, vitamin, and mineral intake in all patients with CKD or ESRD.

Patients on dialysis should *not* follow a standard pre-MBS and post-MBS diet. Instead, the preoperative and postoperative diets should be modified based on the specific individual nephrology needs of that patient.[24] In addition, typical vitamin and mineral supplementation is not recommended for patients with CKD stage 4 or 5 or for patients on dialysis because of the potential nephrotoxicity of vitamins and minerals that are cleared renally, such as vitamin A and magnesium.

Box 7.10 outlines presurgical nutrient recommendations for MBS patients who have CKD. Box 7.11 on page 162 outlines the nutrient needs of patients who have ESRD and are on dialysis. It is very important that the bariatric RDN works with the patient's renal dietitian when designing preoperative and postoperative diets and supplements regimens for these patients.[25] Box 7.12 on page 163 focuses on the nutrition needs of patients who have undergone the RYGB procedure and continue to have ESRD.

BOX 7.10 Nutrient Recommendations for Premetabolic and Bariatric Surgery Patients with Chronic Kidney Disease Stages 1 to 4 and Obesity[a,25]

Nutrient	*Daily recommendations*
Fluids	No restriction Monitor weight gain; should be 2 lb/d or less
Sodium	less than 2.4 g/d
Protein (chronic kidney disease)	Low-protein diet (0.6 to 0.8 g/kg body weight)
Calcium	1,000 to 1,500 mg/d Supplementation recommendations are based on serum calcium levels. If calcium levels are below laboratory normal value, calcium supplementation should be given in the form of oral calcium citrate (1,500 mg/d or less)
Vitamin D	Base supplementation on serum 25-hyroxyvitamin D: • If serum 25-hyroxyvitamin D less than 30 ng/mL, supplement with therapeutic doses of ergocalciferol. If serum phosphorus exceeds 4.6 mg/dL with phosphate binders, discontinue ergocalciferol. • If serum 25-hyroxyvitamin D less than 30 ng/mL, parathyroid hormone is above target range, serum calcium corrected levels less than 9.5 mg/dL, and serum phosphorus more than 4.6 mg/dL, an active oral vitamin D sterol (eg, calcitriol) is indicated.
Iron	325 mg ferrous sulfate three times daily
Potassium	less than 2.4 g/d
Phosphorus	800 to 1,000 mg/d when serum phosphorus more than 4.5 mg
Vitamins B6 and 12, and folate	Dietary reference intake (DRI)
Magnesium	DRI
Zinc	Individualize based on patient's laboratory data

[a] Unless otherwise indicated, recommendations are for total intake (food and supplements). Bariatric registered dietitian nutritionist working with patients who have chronic kidney disease should consult with the patient's renal registered dietitian nutritionist/team regarding diet and supplementation.

BOX 7.11 Nutrient Recommendations for Patients With Obesity and End-Stage Renal Disease on Dialysis[a,25]

Nutrient	***Daily recommendations***
Fluids	Intake = urine output + 1,000 mL
Sodium	Intake less than2.4 g
Protein	1.2 g/kg dry weight
Calcium	Less than2,000 mg, including binders
Vitamin D	Base supplementation on serum 25-hyroxyvitamin D: • If serum 25-hyroxyvitamin D less than30 ng/mL, supplement with therapeutic dose ergocalciferol. If serum phosphorus more than4.5 mg/dL with phosphate binders, discontinue ergocalciferol. • If serum 25-hydroxyvitamin D more than30 ng/mL, parathyroid hormone more thantarget range, serum calcium corrected levels less than9.5 mg/dL, and serum phosphorus less than4.5 mg/dL, an active oral vitamin D sterol (eg, calcitriol) is indicated.
Iron	325 mg ferrous sulfate dietary reference intakeplus additional supplementation until transferrin is more than20% and serum ferritin concentration more than100 or 200 ng/mL
Potassium	Less than2.4 g
Phosphorus	800 to 1,000 mg when serum phosphorus more than5.5 mg[b]
Vitamin C	100 mg orally
Folate	1 mg orally
Vitamin B6	2 mg
Zinc	15 mg

[a]Unless otherwise indicated, recommendations are for total intake (from food and supplements). Bariatric registered dietitian nutritionists working with patients on renal dialysis should consult with the patient's renal registered dietitian nutritionist/team regarding diet and supplementation.

[b]If serum phosphorus 5.5 mg or less, individualize requirement according to patient's laboratory data.

BOX 7.12 Nutrient Recommendations for Post-Roux-en-Y Gastric Bypass Patients With End-Stage Renal Disease[a,b,25]

Nutrient	*Daily recommendations*
Fluids	48 oz or more
Sodium	Less than 2.4 g
Protein	1.2 g/kg ideal body weight[c]
Calcium and vitamin D	1,200 to 1,500 mg[d] oral calcium citrate and 800 IU (20 mcg) of vitamin D daily in a liquid or chewable form
Iron	325 mg ferrous sulfate three times per day[e]
Potassium	Restrict daily intake to less than 2.4 g
Phosphorus	800 to 1,000 mg when serum phosphorus more than 5.5 mg[f]
Vitamin C	Dietary reference intake (DRI)
Folate	400 mcg dietary folate equivalent (DFE)
Vitamin B6	DRI
Zinc	Men: 11 mg Women: 8 mg

[a] Unless otherwise indicated, recommendations are for total intake (from food and supplements). Bariatric registered dietitian nutritionists working with patients on renal dialysis should consult with the patient's renal registered dietitian nutritionist/team regarding diet and supplementation.

[b] Specific recommendations for transgender and gender-diverse people were not provided.

[c] Carefully monitor with chronic kidney disease stages 1 through 4.

[d] The type of calcium recommended for patients on dialysis is calcium acetate. Calcium carbonate is not well absorbed after gastric bypass surgery, and calcium citrate may be contraindicated in patients on dialysis. If patients are taking aluminum-based binders, calcium citrate could increase aluminum toxicity.

[e] More iron may be needed for dialysis loss.

[f] If serum phosphorus 5.5 mg or less, individualize requirement according to patient's laboratory data.

Renal Transplantation

Metabolic and bariatric surgery is more commonly being used as a bridge to renal transplant.[22] Thus, the bariatric RDN is likely to see post–renal transplant patients for long-term bariatric care. Box 7.13[25] lists the nutritional considerations for post-RYGB patients who have undergone a renal transplant. Limited data and recommendations are available for post–sleeve gastrectomy and renal transplant patients. Although undergoing prior MBS is associated with smaller posttransplant weight gain, overall weight gain prevention is a notable challenge.[26]

Kidney Stones

Calcium oxalate stones can form after MBS. The development of these stones is related to hyperoxaluria, low urinary volume, and hypocitraturia.[4]

Patients who have developed oxalate stones or who may be at high risk of stone development should be counseled to do the following:

- Follow a low-fat diet that limits oxalates to 40 to 50 mg/d. Oxalates are found in a wide variety of plant foods and are rare in animal products. High-oxalate foods (higher than 10 mg oxalate per serving), such as nuts, beets, spinach, rhubarb, strawberries, wheat bran, chocolate, and tea, should be avoided.
- Incorporate high-calcium foods into meals (more than 1,000 mg/d) to help bind oxalate before it is absorbed or take a calcium citrate supplement with each meal.
- Avoid dehydration. Increase intake of fluids to 60 to 80 oz/d. Urine should be clear to indicate good fluid status.

Pregnancy

People assigned female at birth undergo more MBS procedures than people assigned male at birth (about 80% are performed on those assigned female at birth); most MBS patients are of reproductive age (18 to 44

BOX 7.13 Nutrient Recommendations for Patients After Roux-en-Y Gastric Bypass and Renal Transplant[a,b,25]

Nutrient	*Daily recommendations*
Fluids	30 to 35 mL/kg ideal body weight
Sodium	No restriction but intake less than 2.4 g is recommended
Protein	1 to 1.2 g/kg ideal body weight
Calcium and vitamin D	1,500 mg calcium[c] or higher plus individualized vitamin D supplementation based on serum vitamin D, parathyroid hormone, and calcium levels
Iron	Dietary reference intake (DRI)
Potassium	No restriction
Phosphorus	No restriction
Vitamin C	DRI
Folate	DRI
Vitamin B6	DRI or higher
Zinc	Men: 11 mg Women: 8 mg
Magnesium	Individualize for immunosuppression loss

[a]Unless otherwise indicated, recommendations are for total intake (from food and supplements). Bariatric registered dietitian nutritionists working with patients on renal dialysis should consult with the patient's renal registered dietitian nutritionist/team regarding diet and supplementation.
[b]Specific recommendations for transgender and gender-diverse people were not provided.
[c]Calcium supplementation is essential to meet daily needs; advise patients to talk with their renal dietitian for a list of appropriate calcium supplements for postoperative supplementation. Since calcium carbonate is not well absorbed after gastric bypass surgery and calcium citrate may be contraindicated in patients on dialysis, the calcium typically recommended is calcium acetate.

years).[27-29] Data on long-term outcomes of MBS for people who give birth and their offspring are needed.[30] Current published data do not include people with multiple gestations after MBS or on revisional surgeries specifically.

Fertility improves after weight loss and bariatric surgery, particularly in people with polycystic ovary syndrome.[31] MBS may be an effective treatment to improve fertility in people with severe obesity through significant and sustained weight loss. However, it is uncertain of the specific impact that MBS has on the responsiveness of subsequent treatments for infertility.[32]

Timing of Pregnancy After Metabolic and Bariatric Surgery

People who have MBS must take precautions against becoming pregnant for at least 12 months after the procedure,[33-35] although people have delivered healthy babies that were conceived in the first year after MBS.[36] However, pregnancy in the early postsurgical period (less than 12 months) may compromise optimal weight outcomes for the parent and present a risk of malnutrition to both parent and fetus. Buchwald and colleagues[27] suggest waiting for up to 2 years after MBS before conceiving. Parent and colleagues[37] also suggest waiting until 2 years post-MBS to give birth. They noted that infants born to people within the 2 years after MBS experienced higher rates of prematurity, neonatal intensive care unit (NICU) admissions, and small-for-gestational-age (SGA) status. Others posit that pregnancy should be delayed until a patient's risk factors are minimized, the patient achieves optimal weight outcomes, and the patient's nutritional deficiencies are identified and treated.[28,36,38-40]

The need to delay pregnancy after MBS can be an important consideration for people who wish to give birth. Therefore, physicians should initiate discussions of contraception and the timing of pregnancy with patients during the *presurgical* consultations. Some people may decide to pursue pregnancy first and then have surgery.

After surgery, discussions of contraception and the timing of pregnancy should be individualized according to the patient's health status and wishes about family planning. The bioavailability of oral contraceptives may be affected after MBS. Schlatter[41] suggests to evaluate with respect to the absorption site, mechanism of absorption, and any other factors that may influence the effectiveness.

Pregnancy Complications Related to Metabolic and Bariatric Surgery

Malnutrition and vitamin/mineral deficiencies can occur at any time (even years) after MBS and could affect parental and fetal outcomes. Thus, regular monitoring and evaluation are important for all pregnancies after MBS.

Pregnant patients with obesity, including after MBS, have significantly higher rates of the following adverse outcomes than do normal-weight pregnant patients:

- gestational hypertension
- preeclampsia
- gestational diabetes mellitus (GDM)
- preterm delivery
- macrosomia (birth weight higher than 4,000 g)
- cesarean sections
- delivery complications

GDM is linked to adverse fetal outcomes.[43] The rate of GDM is lower in pregnant people after MBS than in people with obesity who do not have MBS.[44]

People with obesity after gastric bypass surgery have an increased incidence of fetal growth restriction, SGA infants, and stillbirth.[45] People who become pregnant after biliopancreatic diversion with duodenal switch (BPD/DS), RYGB, and SG are at increased risk of delivering low-birth-weight and SGA infants and should therefore be closely monitored during pregnancy.[31,43,46,47,44,46-48]

In contrast, studies suggest that people with obesity who become pregnant after RYGB, SG, and adjustable gastric banding (AGB) have fewer obesity-related complications than pregnant people with obesity in the general population.[49-51] The incidence of adverse parental and fetal outcomes may approach the rates of people without obesity.[33,52-54]

Compared with their siblings born before MBS, children born to parents after AGB surgery had lower (but appropriate) birth weights and maintained a lower weight over time than their siblings.[33,55-56] Children born to parents after RYGB surgery, compared to siblings born before the MBS procedure, had a lower risk for a high birth weight and increased risk for low birth weight.[57]

Pregnant patients with an AGB should be monitored closely, as band adjustments may be necessary.[33] Surgical complications (eg, slippage of the AGB, intestinal or internal hernias, or bowel obstructions) are potentially serious, especially in pregnancy.[58-59] Symptoms may include abdominal pain or discomfort, nausea, or vomiting—unspecific symptoms that are common in both pregnancy and MBS.[33,34,39]

Nutrition Therapy Goals

Nutrition goals for people who become pregnant after MBS include the following:

- Gain adequate gestational weight to promote fetal growth but reduce the risk of excess weight gain and weight retention (see Box 7.14).[60]
- Receive adequate vitamin and mineral supplementation to correct or prevent deficiencies.
- Receive education on nutrition and hydration during pregnancy and lactation and post–bariatric surgery issues that affect pregnancy.

Nutrition Assessment

Nutrition assessment of pregnant MBS patients should ideally be performed by an RDN who specializes in pregnancy. However, obstetric RDNs who are unfamiliar with MBS procedures should consult with the bariatric RDN.

BOX 7.14 Institute of Medicine Recommendations for Weight Gain During Pregnancy[a,60]

Prepregnancy body mass index 25.0 to 29.0

Recommended total pregnancy weight gain: 7 to 11.5 kg (15 to 25 lb)

Recommended weekly rate of weight gain in second and third trimesters: 0.3 kg (0.6 lb)

Prepregnancy body mass index 30 or higher

Recommended total pregnancy weight gain: 5 to 9 kg (11 to 18 lb)

Recommended weekly rate of weight gain in second and third trimesters: 0.2 kg (0.5 lb)

[a] Institute of Medicine guidelines are based on prepregnant body mass index and do not include specific guidelines for people after bariatric surgery. Recommendations presented here are for singleton pregnancies.

Biochemical Surveillance

To evaluate the client's nutrition-related laboratory values (see Appendix C), the RDN should obtain appropriate reference values from the testing laboratory. Many reference values are specific to pregnancy and may vary by stage of pregnancy.[61,62] The frequency of monitoring depends on the nutritional status of the patient and the pregnancy stage. For more information regarding laboratory reference values for people during pregnancy reference *Williams Obstetrics* laboratory values by trimester.[63]

Patients with GDM require close surveillance. Due to volume restrictions after MBS, patients may not be able to consume the required volume of oral solution within the time period to meet glucose testing guidelines. The oral glucose load may cause dumping syndrome in people with RYGB or BPD/DS. Patients should discuss GDM screening with their physician and consider self-monitoring of blood glucose before and after meals instead. Some of these methods may include 2-hour postprandial testing, continuous glucose monitoring, or a 7-point capillary blood glucose profile.

Food/Nutrition-Related History

Assessment of the pregnant patient's food and nutrient intake should include the following:

- current intake patterns
- energy, protein, and fluid intake
- adherence with supplementation recommendations
- food intolerances
- disordered eating patterns, including pica, food aversions, binge eating, bulimia, or anorexia
- changes in bowel movements and regulation
- review of current laboratory values

Nutrient Supplementation

There is lack of evidence on optimal nutrition monitoring and recommended supplementation during pregnancy after MBS. In a planned pregnancy, nutrient supplementation should be optimized before conception. Guidelines for the nonpregnant post-MBS population are utilized, and pregnancy-specific data should be added where available.[63]

The RDN should assess the patient's vitamin/mineral intake from all sources. Recommendations can then be formulated to meet requirements and avoid possible risks of excess intake.[64]

Anthropometric Measurements

The nutrition assessment should include the following anthropometric data:

- height
- weight
- prepregnancy BMI
- weight change (total loss, percentage of excess weight loss, weight regain) since MBS
- total weight change (loss or gain) and average rate (per week) from start of pregnancy

- weight history from any previous pregnancies (total weight gain, weight retention)

Nutrition-Related Physical Findings

The RDN should assess the patient for the following:

- changes in hair, skin, and nails
- changes in memory (memory lapses)
- numbness or tingling in hands or feet
- burning sensation in feet
- edema
- other signs or symptoms of nutrition-related problems or conditions

Nutrition Diagnosis

The nutrition diagnosis is related to clinical findings of the nutrition evaluation. Examples of possible PES (problem, etiology, signs and symptoms) statements for pregnancy-related etiologies in bariatric patients are listed in Box 7.15 on page 172.[20]

Nutrition Intervention

RDNs working with pregnant patients who have had metabolic and bariatric surgery should refer them to an RDN who specializes in obstetrics. Box 7.16 on pages 172 to 173 lists nutritional requirements for pregnant people who have undergone metabolic and bariatric surgery.[64-67]

Strategies to Increase Energy Intake

For patients with a normal BMI before pregnancy, the general recommendation is to increase energy intake by 340 kcal/d from the third trimester to birth. However, energy requirements may be different for patients with obesity.[74]

BOX 7.15 Selected Nutrition Diagnoses for Pregnant Metabolic and Bariatric Patients

Excessive energy intake related to weight above recommended gestational weight gain targets

Inadequate fluid intake related to increased needs but limited intake or volume tolerance

Excessive alcohol intake

Excessive fat intake

Inadequate vitamin intake (thiamin) related to hyperemesis, which increases risk for thiamin insufficiency during pregnancy beyond the risk generally associated with metabolic and bariatric surgery

Altered gastrointestinal function related to hyperemesis

Inadequate mineral intake (iron)

Overweight/obesity

Unintended weight gain

Food- and nutrition-related knowledge deficit

Not ready for diet/lifestyle change

Disordered eating pattern

Undesirable food choices

Physical inactivity

Inability to manage self-care

BOX 7.16 Sample Nutrition Prescription for a Pregnant Patient After Metabolic and Bariatric Surgery[64-73]

Energy	Energy should be adequate to achieve gestational weight gain targets and optimize fetal growth.
Protein	1.2 g/kg of ideal body weight
	Oral protein supplements may be required.
Fluid	Total fluid = 3 L (6 oz) per day
	Avoid alcohol and energy drinks.

BOX 7.16	Sample Nutrition Prescription for a Pregnant Patient After Metabolic and Bariatric Surgery[64-73] (cont.)
Omega-3 fatty acids	Dietary source of docosahexaenoic acid (DHA) is desirable: at least two servings per week of cooked fish that is low in mercury and high in omega-3 fatty acids. Consider a DHA supplement if consuming less than the recommended amount of fish.
Vitamin and mineral supplementation	To prevent deficiency, meet additional needs of pregnancy, and to optimize fetal growth, single-format supplements (eg, iron, folic acid, vitamin D, vitamin B12) should be considered in addition to the bariatric vitamin regimen.
Folic acid	People at risk of folate deficiency (BMI higher than 35, those with diabetes, malabsorptive procedures or disorders, suboptimal adherence to supplements, or those with a history of prior pregnancies complicated by neural tube defects) should take 5 mg/d for 2 months before pregnancy and the first 12 weeks of the pregnancy. After the first 12 weeks, supplement folic acid according to standard pregnancy guidelines (0.4 to 1.0 mg/d) for rest of the pregnancy and at least 4 to 6 weeks postpartum or for the duration of breastfeeding.[68] Recently, some guidelines discontinued using the 5 mg dosage of folic acid due to concerns about possible excess supplementation with consideration of intake of folate-fortified foods.[70]
Vitamin A	Both vitamin A excess and deficiency are associated with birth defects. The recommended upper limit for retinol supplements is 5,000 IU/d (1,500 mcg), but higher doses (eg, 8,000 to 10,000 IU/d [2,400 to 3,000 mcg/d]) have not been found to be associated with increased risk of fetal malformations. These recommendations are not specific to the metabolic and bariatric surgerypopulation; upper limits have not been established for vitamin A during pregnancy in this group. Therefore, there is conflicting data on repletion recommendations and the use of retinol during pregnancy. It is suggested to use β carotene during pregnancy and not to utilize retinol after the first days of gestation.[71,72]
Choline	The recommended amount of choline during pregnancy is 450 mg. In 2017, the American Medical Association supported an increase in prenatal vitamins to ensure this recommendation. An additional supplement may need to be given to meet this recommendation.[73]

If pregnant patients struggle to achieve their recommended energy intake goal because of limited gastric capacity, the following practices may help:

- Eat five or six small meals or snacks each day.
- Include a protein choice with each meal or snack to help meet requirements.
- Choose at least 2 cups of fluid milk or a fortified plant-based beverage (note that soy-based beverages are higher in protein than nut- or rice-based drinks).
- Avoid consuming liquids with meals.
- Choose nutrient-dense foods.

Consider nutrition support for patients who are unable to meet goals regarding gestational weight gain, weight loss, or fetal growth. Oral protein supplements may be appropriate for some patients, especially if weight gain targets are not met or pregnancy occurs less than 12 months after surgery.[28]

Patients who experience recurrent nausea and vomiting, abdominal pain, or low gestational weight gain should be assessed by a bariatric surgeon for possible surgical complications.[27,28,75]

Nutrition Education and Counseling

Nutrition education and counseling is a critical part of prenatal care. For more information about education and counseling refer to Appendix H. Topics for nutrition education and counseling for pregnant MBS patients include the following:

- gestational weight gain targets
- nutrient and fluid requirements of pregnancy, including vitamin and mineral supplementation
- food and drinks not recommended in pregnancy
- food safety
- management of common complications
- lactation and breastfeeding
- realistic postpartum weight goals

Collaboration and Referral of Care

Care for patients who are pregnant after MBS is complex and requires support and services beyond the scope of dietetics practice. The following providers should be part of the multidisciplinary health care team:

- primary care physician/provider
- obstetrician with experience in high-risk pregnancies
- obstetric internist (internal medicine specialist) with expertise in caring for medical problems
- bariatric surgeon
- lactation consultant to support breastfeeding
- pharmacist
- mental health provider
- RDNs with expertise in pregnancy, lactation, metabolic and bariatric surgery, and pediatrics

Nutrition Monitoring and Evaluation

The RDN should monitor the following in people who are pregnant after MBS[20]:

- Body composition/growth/weight history—weight change
  - weight gain
  - weight change percentage
  - weight change intent
  - measured gestational weight gain
- Behavior—adherence
  - nutrition self-monitoring at agreed-upon rate
  - self-reported nutrition adherence score
- Intake
  - caffeinated beverage estimated oral intake in 24 hours
  - water measured oral intake in 24 hours
  - protein food servings measured in 24 hours

- Nutrition-focused physical findings
  - digestive system
    - nausea
    - vomiting
    - constipation
  - hair—hair changes due to malnutrition
  - nails
    - pail nail bed
    - koilonychia
    - leukonychia
    - micronutrient intake
  - vitamin intake—multivitamin measured intake in 24 hours
  - mineral intake
    - chromium estimated intake in 24 hours
    - iron estimated intake in 24 hours

MBSis being established as a treatment option for more populations, increasing the number of people who choose surgery as their primary treatment option and diversifying the concurrent medical nutrition therapy needs of the surgical population. Special considerations in surgical obesity treatment have been and will likely continue to be ever-evolving. Although the information presented in the chapter provides a comprehensive review of the recommendations for endocrine-related and kidney-related diagnoses as well as pregnancy, RDNs are responsible for continuing to stay abreast of emerging data, potentially contributing to the literature and collaborating with other subspecialized clinicians as a standard of practice. Of particular importance, RDNs can use this guidance coupled with emerging evidence and patient-centered education and counseling (Appendix H) to assist these individuals in reaching their health goals while managing multiple considerations.

References

1. Eisenberg D, Azagury DE, Ghiassi S, Grover BT, Kim JJ. ASMBS position statement on postprandial hyperinsulinemic hypoglycemia after MBS. *Surg Obes Relat Dis*. 2017;(3):371. doi:10.1016/j.soard.2016.12.005
2. Suhl E, Anderson-Haynes S-E, Mulla C, Patti M-E. Medical nutrition therapy for post-bariatric hypoglycemia: practical insights. *Surg Obes Relat Dis*. 2017;13(5):888-896. doi:10.1016/j.soard.2017.01.025
3. Nor Hanipah Z, Punchai S, Birriel TJ, et al. Clinical features of symptomatic hypoglycemia observed after bariatric surgery. *Surg Obes Relat Dis*. 2018;14(9):1335-1339. doi:10.1016/j.soard.2018.02.022
4. Tack J, Arts J, Caenepeel P, De Wulf D, Bisschops R. Pathophysiology, diagnosis and management of postoperative dumping syndrome. *Nat Rev Gastroenty Hepatol*. 2009;6(10):583. doi:10.1038/nrgastro.2009.148
5. de Heide LJM, Glaudemans AWJM, Oomen PHN, Apers JA, Totte ERE, van Beek AP. Functional imaging in hyperinsulinemic hypoglycemia after gastric bypass surgery for morbid obesity. *J Clin Endocrinol Metab*. 2012;97(6):E963-E967.
6. Patti ME, McMahon G, Mun EC, et al. Severe hypoglycaemia post-gastric bypass requiring partial pancreatectomy: evidence for inappropriate insulin secretion and pancreatic islet hyperplasia. *Diabetologia*. 2005;48(11):2236-2240. doi:10.1007/s00125-005-1933-x
7. Kellogg TA, Bantle JP, Leslie DB, et al. Postgastric bypass hyperinsulinemic hypoglycemia syndrome: characterization and response to a modified diet. *Surg Obes Relat Dis*. 2008;4(4):492-499. doi:10.1016/j.soard.2008.05.005
8. Moreira RO, Moreira RB, Machado NA, Goncalves TB, Coutinho WF. Post-prandial hypoglycemia after bariatric surgery: pharmacological treatment with verapamil and acarbose. *Obes Surg*. 2008;18(12):1618. doi:10.1007/s11695-008-9569-9
9. Z'graggen K, Guwedhi A, Steffan R, et al. Severe recurrent hypoglycemia after gastric bypass surgery. *Obes Surg*. 2008;18(8):981. doi:10.1007/s11695-008-9480-4
10. Dapri G, Cadière GB, Himpens J. Laparoscopic reconversion of Roux-en-Y gastric bypass to original anatomy: technique and preliminary outcomes. *Obes Surg*. 2011;21(8):1289-1295. doi:10.1007/s11695-010-0252-6
11. Chillarón JJ, Flores Le-Roux JA, Benaiges D, Pedro-Botet J. Type 1 diabetes, metabolic syndrome and cardiovascular risk. *Metabolism*. 2014;63(2):181-187. doi:10.1016/j.metabol.2013.10.002

12. Corbin KD, Driscoll KA, Pratley RE, et al. Obesity in type 1 diabetes: pathophysiology, clinical impact, and mechanisms. *Endocr Rev.* 2018;39(5):629-663. doi:10.1210/er.2017-00191
13. Yeung KTD, Reddy M, Purkayastha S. Surgical options for glycaemic control in type 1 diabetes. *Diabet Med.* 2019;36(4):414-423. doi:10.1111/dme.13885
14. Rottenstreich A, Keidar A, Yuval JB, Abu-gazala M, Khalaileh A, Elazary R. Outcome of bariatric surgery in patients with type 1 diabetes mellitus: our experience and review of the literature. *Surg Endosc.* 2016;30(12):5428-5433. doi:10.1007/s00464-016-4901-2
15. Czupryniak L, Wiszniewski M, Szymanski D, Pawlowski M, Loba J, Strzelczyk J. Long-term results of gastric bypass surgery in morbidly obese type 1 diabetes patients. *Obes Surg.* 2010;20(4):506-508. doi:10.1007/s11695-010-0074-6
16. Mendez CE, Tanenberg RJ, Pories W. Outcomes of Roux-en-Y gastric bypass surgery for severely obese patients with type 1 diabetes: a case series report. *Diabetes Metab Syndr Obes.* 2010;3:281-283.
17. Vilarrasa N, Rubio MA, Miñambres I, et al. Long-term outcomes in patients with morbid obesity and type 1 diabetes undergoing bariatric surgery. *Obes Surg.* 2017;27(4):856-863. doi:10.1007/s11695-016-2390-y
18. American Diabetes Association. Standards of medical care in diabetes. *Diabetes Care.* 2019;42(suppl):S46-S71.
19. Dowsett J, Humphreys R, Krones R. Normal blood glucose and high blood ketones in a critically unwell patient with T1DM post-bariatric surgery: a case of euglycemic diabetic ketoacidosis. *Obes Surg.* 2019;29(1):347-349. doi:10.1007/s11695-018-3548-6
20. Academy of Nutrition and Dietetics. Nutrition terminology reference manual (eNCPT): dietetics language for nutrition care. Accessed June 26, 2020. http://ncpt.webauthor.com
21. Bilha SC, Nistor I, Nedelcu A, et al. The effects of bariatric surgery on renal outcomes: a systematic review and meta-analysis. *Obes Surg.* 2018;28(12):3815-3833. doi:10.1007/s11695-018-3416-4
22. Bouchard P, Tchervenkov J, Demyttenaere S, Court O, Andalib A. Safety and efficacy of the sleeve gastrectomy as a strategy towards kidney transplantation. *Surg Endosc.* 2020;34(6):2657-2664. doi:10.1007/s00464-019-07042-z
23. Takata MC, Campos GM, Ciovica R, et al. Laparoscopic bariatric surgery improves candidacy in morbidly obese patients awaiting transplantation. *Surg Obes Relat Dis.* 2008;4(2):159-164. doi:10.1016/j.soard.2007.12.009
24. Ben-Porat T, Weiss-Sadan A, Rottenstreich A, et al. Nutritional management for chronic kidney disease patients who undergo bariatric surgery: a narrative review. *Adv Nutr.* 2019;10(1):122-132. doi:10.1093/advances/nmy112

25. Lightner AL, Lau J, Obayashi P, Birge K, Melcher ML. Potential nutritional conflicts in bariatric and renal transplant patients. *Obes Surg.* 2011;21(12):1965-1970. doi:10.1007/s11695-011-0423-0
26. Cohen JB, Lim MA, Tewksbury CM, et al. Bariatric surgery before and after kidney transplantation: long-term weight loss and allograft outcomes. *Surg Obes Relat Dis.* 2019;15(6):935-941. doi:10.1016/j.soard.2019.04.002
27. Buchwald H, Avidor Y, Braunwald E, et al. Bariatric surgery: a systematic review and meta-analysis. *JAMA.* 2004;292(14):1724-1737. doi:10.1001/jama.292.14.1724
28. Patel JA, Colella JJ, Esaka E, Patel NA, Thomas RL. Improvement in infertility and pregnancy outcomes after weight loss surgery. *Med Clin N Am.* 2007;91(3):515-528. doi:10.1016/j.mcna.2007.01.002
29. Healthgrades. 2015 bariatric surgery analysis gender-related differences in obesity, complications and risks. Accessed September 2, 2019. www.healthgrades.com/quality/2015-healthgrades-bariatric-surgery-white-paper
30. Kominiarek MA. Pregnancy after bariatric surgery. *Obstet Gynecol Clin N Am.* 2010;37(2):305-320. doi:10.1016/j.ogc.2010.02.010
31. Agency for Health Care Research and Quality. Bariatric surgery in women of reproductive age: special considerations for pregnancy. Evidence Report/Technology Assessment no. 169. November 2008. Accessed March 11, 2014. www.ahrq.gov/research/findings/evidence-based-reports/er169-abstract.html
32. Sheiner E, Willis K, Yogev Y. Bariatric surgery: impact on pregnancy outcomes. *Curr Diab Rep.* 2012;13(1):19-26. doi:10.1007/s11892-012-0329-9
33. Maggard MA, Yermilov I, Li Z, et al. Pregnancy and fertility following bariatric surgery: a systematic review. *JAMA.* 2008;300(19):2286-2296. doi:10.1001/jama.2008.641
34. Guelinckx I, Devlieger R, Vansant G. Reproductive outcome after bariatric surgery: a critical review. *Hum Reprod Update.* 2009;15(2):189-201. doi:10.1093/humupd/dmn057
35. Magdaleno R Jr, Pereira BG, Chaim EA, Turato ER. Pregnancy after bariatric surgery: a current view of maternal, obstetrical and perinatal challenges. *Arch Gynecol Obstet.* 2011;285(3):559-566. doi:10.1007/s00404-011-2187-0
36. Dao T, Kuhn J, Ehmer D, Fisher T, McCarty T. Pregnancy outcomes after gastric bypass surgery. *Am J Surg.* 2006;192(6):762-766. doi:10.1016/j.amjsurg.2006.08.041
37. Parent B, Martopullo I, Weiss NS, Khandelwal S, Fay EE, Rowhani-Rahbar A. Bariatric surgery in women of childbearing age, timing between an operation and birth, and associated perinatal complications. *JAMA Surg.* 2017;152(2):128. doi:10.1001/jamasurg.2016.3621

38. American Dietetic Association; American Society of Nutrition; Siega-Riz AM, King JC. Position of the American Dietetic Association and American Society for Nutrition: obesity, reproduction, and pregnancy outcomes. *J Am Diet Assoc.* 2009;109(5):918-927. doi:10.1016/j.jada.2009.03.020

39. Sheiner E, Edri A, Balaban E, Levi I, Aricha-Tamir B. Pregnancy outcome of patients who conceive during or after the first year following bariatric surgery. *Am J Obstet Gynecol.* 2011;204(1):50.e1-50.e506. doi:10.1016/j.ajog.2010.08.027

40. Mechanick JI, Kushner RF, Sugerman HJ, et al. American Association of Clinical Endocrinologists, the Obesity Society, and American Society for Metabolic & Bariatric Surgery medical guidelines for clinical practice for the perioperative nutritional, metabolic, and nonsurgical support of the bariatric surgery patient. *Obesity.* 2009;17 suppl 1:S1-70, v. doi:10.1038/oby.2009.28

41. Schlatter J. Oral contraceptives after bariatric surgery. *Obes Facts.* 2017;10(2):118-126. doi:10.1159/000449508

42. Nuthalapaty FS, Rouse DJ. The impact of obesity on obstetrical practice and outcome. *Clin Obestet Gynecol.* 2004;47(4):898-981. doi:10.1097/01.grf.0000135358.34673.48

43. Rundra CB, Sorensen TK, Leisenring WM, Dashow E, Williams MA. Weight characteristic and height in relation to risk of gestational diabetes mellitus. *Am J Epidemiol.* 2007;165(3):302-308. doi:10.1093/aje/kwk007

44. Badreldin N, Kuller J, Rhee E, Brown L, Laifer S. Pregnancy management after bariatric surgery. *Obstet Gynecol Surv.* 2016;71(6):361-368. doi:10.1097/OGX.0000000000000322

45. Lesko J, Peaceman A. Pregnancy outcomes in women after bariatric surgery compared with obese and morbidly obese controls. *Obstet Gynecol.* 2012;119(3):547-554. doi:10.1097/AOG.0b013e318239060e

46. Friedman D, Cuneo S, Valenzano M, et al. Pregnancies in an 18-year follow up after biliopancreatic diversion. *Obes Surg.* 1995;5:308-313. doi:10.1381/096089295765557692

47. Rottenstreich A, Elchalal U, Kleinstern G, Beglaibter N, Khalaileh A, Elazary R. Maternal and perinatal outcomes after laparoscopic sleeve gastrectomy. *Obstet Gynecol.* 2018;131(3):451-456. doi:10.1097/AOG.0000000000002481

48. Santulli P, Mandelbrot L, Facchiano E, et al. Obstetrical and neonatal outcomes of pregnancies following gastric bypass surgery: a retrospective cohort study in a french referral centre. *Obes Surg.* 2010;20(11):1501-1508. doi:10.1007/s11695-010-0260-6

49. Wittgrove AC, Jester L, Wittgrove P, Clark GW. Pregnancy following gastric bypass for morbid obesity. *Obes Surg.* 1998;8(4):461-466. doi:10.1381/096089298765554368

50. Dixon JB, Dixon ME, O'Brien PE. Birth outcomes in obese women after laparoscopic adjustable gastric banding. *Obstet Gynecol*. 2005;106(5 Pt 1):965-972. doi:10.2097/01.AOG.0000181821.82022.82
51. Ducarme G, Chesnoy V, Lemarié P, Koumaré S, Krawczykowski D. Pregnancy outcomes after laparoscopic sleeve gastrectomy among obese patients. *Int J Gynecol Obstet*. 2015;130(2):127-131. doi:10.1016/j.ijgo.2015.03.022
52. Sheiner E, Levy A, Silverberg D, et al. Pregnancy after bariatric surgery is not associated with adverse perinatal outcome. *Am J Obstet Gynecol*. 2004;190(5):1335-1340. doi:10.1016/j.ajog.2003.11.004
53. Bennett WL, Gilson MM, Jamshidi R, et al. Impact of bariatric surgery on hypertensive disorders in pregnancy: a retrospective analysis of insurance claims data. *BMJ*. 2010;340:c1662. doi:10.1136/bmj.c1662
54. Burke AE, Bennett WL, Jamshidi RM, et al. Reduced incidence of gestational diabetes with bariatric surgery. *J Am Coll Surg*. 2010;211(2):169-175. doi:10.1016/j.jamcollsurg.2010.03.029
55. Kral JG, Biron S, Simard S, et al. Large maternal weight loss from obesity surgery prevents transmission of obesity to children who were followed for 2 to 18 years. *Pediatrics*. 2006;118(6):e1644-e1649. doi:10.1542/peds.2006-1379
56. Smith J, Cianflone K, Biron S, et al. Effects of maternal surgical weight loss in mothers on intergenerational transmission of obesity. *J Clin Endocrinol Metab*. 2009;94(11):4275-4283. doi:10.1210/jc.2009-0709
57. Adams TD, Hammoud AO, Davidson LE, et al. Maternal and neonatal outcomes for pregnancies before and after gastric bypass surgery. *Int J Obes (Lond)*. 2015;39(4):686-694. doi:10.1038/ijo.2015.9
58. Davis E, Olson C. Obesity in pregnancy. *Prim Care*. 2009;36(2):341-356. doi:10.1016/j.pop.2009.01.005
59. Kakarla N, Dailey C, Marino T, Shikora SA, Chelmow D. Pregnancy after gastric bypass surgery and internal hernia formation. *Obstet Gynecol*. 2005;105(5 Pt 2):1195-1198. doi:10.1097/01.AOG.0000152352.58688.27
60. Rasmussen KM, Yaktine AL; Institute of Medicine (US) Committee to Reexamine IOM Pregnancy Weight Guidelines, eds. *Weight Gain During Pregnancy: Reexamining the Guidelines*. National Academies Press (US); 2009.
61. Blankenship JD, Turnier-Lamoureaux N. Pregnancy 101: laboratory assessment. *Women's Health Reprod Nutr Rep*. 2005:5;6-7.
62. Larsson A, Palm M, Hansson LO, Axelsson O. Reference values for clinical chemistry tests during normal pregnancy. *BJOG*. 2008;115(7):874-881. doi:10.1111/j.1471-0528.2008.01709.x
63. Cunningham FG, Levano KJ, Bloom SL. *Williams Obstetrics*. 25th ed. Mcgraw-Hill Education, Inc; 2018.

64. National Institute of Medicine. *Dietary Reference Intakes for Water, Potassium, Chloride, and Sulfate*. National Academies Press; 2004.

65. American College of Obstetricians and Gynecologists. ACOG practice bulletin no. 105: bariatric surgery and pregnancy. *Obstet Gynecol.* 2009;113(6):1405-1413. doi:10.1097/AOG.0b013e3181ac0544

66. Wilson RD; Genetics Committee; Motherisk. Pre-conceptional vitamin/folic acid supplementation 2007: the use of folic acid in combination with a multivitamin supplement for the prevention of neural tube defects and other congenital anomalies. *J Obstet Gynaecol Can.* 2007;29(12):1003-1013. doi:10.1016/S1701-2163(16)32685-8

67. Kennedy D, Koren G. Identifying women who might benefit from higher doses of folic acid in pregnancy. *Can Fam Physician.* 2012;58(4):394-397.

68. Slater C, Morris L, Ellison J, Syed A. Nutrition in pregnancy following bariatric surgery. *Nutrients*. 2017;9(12):1338. doi:10.3390/nu9121338

69. Nutrition Working Group; O'Connor DL, Blake J, Bell R, et al. Canadian consensus on female nutrition: adolescence, reproduction, menopause, and beyond. *J Obstet Gynaecol Can.* 2016;38(6):508-554.e18. doi:10.1016/j.jogc.2016.01.001

70. Lamers Y, Macfarlane AJ, O'Connor DL, Fontaine-Bisson B. Periconceptional intake of folic acid among low-risk women in Canada: summary of a workshop aiming to align prenatal folic acid supplement composition with current expert guidelines. *Am J Clin Nutr.* 2018;108(6):1357-1368. doi:10.1093/ajcn/nqy212

71. Vitamin A supplementation during pregnancy. World Health Organization. Accessed March 24, 2020. www.who.int/elena/titles/guidance_summaries/vitamina_pregnancy/en/

72. Shawe J, Ceulemans D, Akhter Z, et al. Pregnancy after bariatric surgery: consensus recommendations for periconception, antenatal and postnatal care. *Obes Rev.* 2019;20(11):1507-1522. doi:10.1111/obr.12927

73. AMA backs global health experts in calling infertility a disease. American Medical Association. Published June 13, 2017. Accessed March 24, 2020. www.ama-assn.org/delivering-care/public-health/ama-backs-global-health-experts-calling-infertility-disease

74. Butte NF, King JC. Energy requirements during pregnancy and lactation. *Pub Health Nutr.* 2005;8(7A):1010-1027. doi:10.1079/phn2005793

75. Moore KA, Ouyang DW, Whang EE. Maternal and fetal deaths after gastric bypass surgery for morbid obesity. *N Engl J Med.* 2004;351(7):721-722. doi:10.1056/NEJM200408123510722

CHAPTER 8

Nutrition Support Therapy After Metabolic and Bariatric Surgery

Metabolic and bariatric surgery (MBS) patients may require nutrition support therapy if they cannot take oral nutrition or have limited gastrointestinal (GI) tract function. The decision process regarding nutrition support in MBS patients follows the same guidelines used for all patients, but special consideration should be given to the challenges of obtaining enteral access after MBS and the unique micronutrient needs of this patient population.

Indications for Nutrition Support

Common GI indications for initiation of nutrition support therapy in the MBS patient are anastomotic leak, fistula, intractable nausea and vomiting, severe malabsorption, diarrhea, and malnutrition (see also Box 8.1 on page 184).[1-5] Other complications that may prompt initiation of nutrition support therapy include ileus, anastomotic stricture, or intestinal obstruction.[2]

BOX 8.1 Indications for Nutrition Support in Metabolic and Bariatric Surgery Patients[1,2,5]

When to use enteral nutrition

Inability to take oral nutrition for more than 7 to 10 days (or for more than 5 to 7 days in intensive care unit setting); must have functional gastrointestinal tract and ability to safely insert an enteral feeding tube

Presence of an enterocutaneous fistula where an enteral feeding tube can be inserted distal to the fistula

Inadequate oral intake to meet metabolic demands (eg, trauma, burn, or other critically ill patients)

Significant malnutrition that cannot be resolved with oral nutritional supplements

When to use parenteral nutrition

Inability to take oral or enteral nutrition for more than 7 to 10 days (or for more than 5 to 7 days in intensive care unit setting)

Diffuse peritonitis

Presence of an enterocutaneous fistula where an enteral feeding tube cannot be inserted distal to the fistula

Gastrointestinal ischemia

Ileus

Intestinal obstruction

Intractable vomiting

Intractable diarrhea

Perioperative nutrition (parenteral nutrition for 7 to 10 days) for severely malnourished patients

Severe malabsorption

Significant malnutrition with inability to obtain enteral access, contraindication to enteral nutrition, or poor tolerance to enteral nutrition

Short bowel syndrome (severe cases)

When a patient is unable to take oral nutrition but otherwise has a functional GI tract, enteral nutrition (EN) is the preferred method of nutrition support therapy.[1] Parenteral nutrition (PN) should be reserved for patients who cannot be enterally fed or who fail an EN trial.[2] Review of the patient's current history and discussion with the surgeon regarding GI function and ability to access the GI tract guide the decision regarding EN or PN (see Box 8.2 on page 186).

Nutrition Assessment

Box 8.3 on page 187 summarizes important factors to evaluate in the nutrition assessment.[1-3,6]

Energy Requirements

Indirect Calorimetry vs Predictive Equations

The optimal method for determining energy requirements in the MBS patient who may need nutrition support is indirect calorimetry.[7] Predictive equations may also be used, but they may overestimate or underestimate energy requirements for patients with obesity and those who have experienced massive weight loss because of their altered body composition. Box 8.4 on page 188 lists equations to determine energy requirements recommended by the Academy of Nutrition and Dietetics Evidence Analysis Library (EAL) Working Group, American Society for Parenteral and Enteral Nutrition (ASPEN), and the Society of Critical Care Medicine.[5,8-12]

Hypocaloric Feeding

Hypocaloric feeding may minimize complications associated with overfeeding, such as hyperglycemia or excessive carbon dioxide production, and may continue to promote weight loss while providing adequate protein to support healing and preservation of lean body mass. In studies evaluating the effectiveness of hypocaloric feeding in hospitalized patients with obesity, high protein delivery (1.5 g/kg or higher ideal

BOX 8.2 Advantages and Disadvantages of Enteral and Parenteral Nutrition[1,2,5]

Enteral nutrition

Advantages:

Preserved intestinal integrity and gut-associated lymphoid tissue (GALT)

Improved glycemic management

Decreased infectious complications

Cost-effective

Disadvantages:

Potential for gastronintestinal (GI) intolerance including nausea, vomiting, abdominal distention, diarrhea, constipation

Risk of aspiration

Difficulty in obtaining enteral access in the metabolic and bariatric surgery patient because of altered GI anatomy

Parenteral nutrition

Advantages:

Able to reliably meet 100% of energy, protein, vitamin, and mineral needs

Relatively easier to obtain access compared with enteral

Able to provide nutrition when enteral feeding is contraindicated

No risk of aspiration related to nutrition support intervention

Disadvantages:

Increased risk of infectious complications

Risk of mechanical complications associated with central venous access

In the long term, may lead to intestinal atrophy, parenteral nutrition–associated liver disease, and metabolic bone disease

High cost

BOX 8.3 Nutrition Assessment of Metabolic and Bariatric Surgery Patients Who May Require Nutrition Support[1-3,6]

Food/nutrition-related history

Diet history with a focus on food and fluid tolerance/intolerance

Ability to take/tolerate vitamin/mineral supplements

Ability to obtain, prepare, and consume food/fluids

Biochemical data, medical tests, and procedures

Studies of electrolytes, circulating proteins, complete blood count, micronutrient levels

Imaging, such as abdominal flat-plate x-ray and abdominal/pelvic computerized tomography scan

Gastric emptying studies, motility studies

Operative notes

Anthropometric measurements

Height

Weight, weight history

Weight change: percentage of total body weight lost and time frame

Body mass index

Nutrition-focused physical findings[a]

Hair quality (coarse, thinning, easily plucked)

Cheilosis

Skin turgor, rashes, open/poorly healing wounds or skin breakdown

Nail quality (brittle, easily broken, koilonychia)

Edema

Fat wasting

Muscle wasting

Client history

Any relevant social or medical history that would impact nutrition support decisions

Outpatient bariatric registered dietitian's assessment, if applicable

[a] Refer to Appendix D for more information.

BOX 8.4 Estimating Resting Metabolic Rate in Patients With Obesity[a,b,5,8-12]

2003 Penn State University (PSU) equation

$$\text{Resting metabolic rate} = (\text{Harris-Benedict} \times 0.85) + (T_{max} \times 175) + (VE \times 33) - 6{,}433$$

where Harris-Benedict is resting metabolic rate (RMR) estimated with the Harris-Benedict equation; T_{max}, maximum body temperature (degrees Celsius) in the previous 24 hours; VE, minute ventilation (L/min). Note: Adjusted weight for obesity is used for patients more than 25% above ideal body weight.

American Society for Parenteral and Enteral Nutrition/Society of Critical Care Medicine guidelines for permissive underfeeding the critically ill patient with obesity

Body mass index (BMI) = 30 to 50: 11 to 14 kcal/kg actual weight

BMI more than 50: 22 to 25 kcal/kg ideal body weight

American Society for Parenteral and Enteral Nutrition clinical guidelines: nutrition support of hospitalized adult patients with obesity

For noncritically ill hospitalized patients with obesity, use the Mifflin-St. Jeor (MSJ) equation:

$$\text{Male: RMR} = (10 \times \text{weight in kg}) + (6.25 \times \text{height in cm}) - (5 \times \text{age in years}) + 5$$

$$\text{Female: RMR} = (10 \times \text{weight in kg}) + (6.25 \times \text{height in cm}) - (5 \times \text{age in years}) - 161$$

For critically ill patients with obesity, age less than 60 years, use the 2010 PSU equation:

$$\text{RMR} = (\text{MSJ} \times 0.96) + (T_{max} \times 167) + (VE \times 31) - 6{,}212$$

For critically ill patients with obesity, age 60 years or higher, use the modified PSU equation:

$$\text{RMR} = (\text{MSJ} \times 0.71) + (T_{max} \times 85) + (VE \times 64) - 3{,}085$$

where MSJ, Mifflin-St. Jeor equation; T_{max}, maximum temperature (degrees Celsius) in the prior 24 hours; VE, minute ventilation (L/min).

[a] Clinicians may use an activity factor (not included here) to estimate total energy requirements.

[b] Specific recommendations for transgender and gender-diverse people were not provided.

body weight) promoted positive nitrogen balance and spared lean body mass.[10,11] These studies are the basis of protein guidelines for the hypocaloric feeding of critically ill patients with obesity.[5]

Protein Requirements

Protein requirements are difficult to determine in patients after MBS. Complicated patients require more than the general recommendation of 60 g/d.[3] The protein requirements for patients who have complications after MBS are not as well defined. Continuous renal replacement therapies, large wounds, and other clinical situations can increase protein demand.[5] The appropriate weight to use to assess protein requirements has not been defined. Box 8.5 on page 190 provides some suggested protein guidelines based on clinical scenarios.[5,12] Refer to Appendix G for discussion of protein-energy malnutrition.

Fluid Requirements

The appropriate weight to use in calculating fluid requirements has not been defined. There are no clear recommendations on whether actual weight, ideal body weight, or another weight should be used for these calculations. See Box 8.6 on page 194 for a general guideline regarding fluid requirements for MBS patients.[3,13] The registered dietitian nutritionist (RDN) should individualize fluid recommendations for patients based on clinical parameters. For example, patients with heart failure or kidney impairment may require a fluid restriction. Patients with severe vomiting, diarrhea, or high-output enterocutaneous fistula may require more fluid to replace losses. Close monitoring of intake/output records correlated with a patient's weight change may help determine if a patient needs an increase or decrease in fluid delivery. The physical examination is also helpful in evaluating hydration status. A patient with a dry mouth or poor skin turgor (eg, "tenting" of skin on examination) may be showing signs of dehydration. Patients with an increase in edema on physical examination may be volume overloaded. Laboratory monitoring can also be helpful; hypernatremia or an elevated blood urea

BOX 8.5 Typical Daily Protein Requirements for Patients Receiving Nutrition Support Therapy[5,12]

Clinical scenario	*Typical protein requirements*
Protein-energy malnutrition, wound healing/hypercatabolism	1.2 to 1.5 g/kg[a]
Continuous renal replacement therapy	1.5 to 2.5 g/kg[a]
Hypocaloric feeding, critically ill patient with class I or class II obesity	2 g/kg or more ideal body weight[b]
Hypocaloric feeding, critically ill patient with class III obesity	2.5 g/kg or more ideal body weight

[a] There is no consensus regarding use of actual body weight vs ideal body weight for this estimate.

[b] There are many ways to determine ideal body weight; clinicians should determine which method is best for their institution and patient population.

BOX 8.6 Methods for Estimating Fluid Requirements for Metabolic and Bariatric Surgery Patients on Nutrition Support[a,3,13]

Typical post–bariatric surgery requirements:

- 1.5 to 1.9 L/d
- 1 mL/kcal

[a] Other methods based on body weight are available for estimating requirements; however, research on their use in patients with obesity is not available.

nitrogen:creatinine ratio may suggest dehydration and hyponatremia may suggest volume overload. Clinical correlation of the intake/output records, weight changes, physical examination, and laboratory values are important in determining volume status and need for change in fluid delivery.[13] See Monitoring and Evaluation on page 197 for more information on clinical parameters to consider when monitoring the patient.

Micronutrient Assessment and Repletion

Assessment and repletion recommendations for micronutrient deficiencies are listed in Appendix D. An MBS patient beginning nutrition support because of severe vomiting has a high risk of thiamin deficiency and Wernicke encephalopathy.[14] If there is concern for Wernicke encephalopathy, there are varying recommendations depending on severity of symptoms as well as the patient's ability to tolerate oral/enteral repletion. For patients who can receive oral or enteral repletion, 100 mg thiamin two to three times per day can be provided until symptoms resolve. For patients with signs of severe deficiency, recommended doses range from 200 mg thiamin intravenously three times per day to 500 mg thiamin once or twice per day for 3 to 5 days, then taper to 250 mg once per day for 3 to 5 days or until symptoms resolve. Patients who have had symptomatic deficiency should continue to receive 100 mg thiamin daily until risk factors for Wernicke encephalopathy (eg, severe vomiting) resolve.[3]

ASPEN has recently published consensus recommendations for refeeding syndrome. Refeeding syndrome is defined as a range of metabolic and electrolyte alterations occurring as a result of the reintroduction or increased provision of calories after a period of decreased or no caloric intake. Refeeding syndrome may be poorly recognized in MBS patients because clinicians may think this syndrome only occurs in underweight patients. This consensus paper highlights many patient populations at risk for refeeding syndrome (including anorexia nervosa, mental health disorders with poor intake, alcohol and substance use disorders, and others) and have a section that includes MBS and bowel resection patients (grouped together for discussion). The authors emphasize that refeeding syndrome can occur regardless of BMI and highlight that patients with obesity can develop malnutrition as with any other patient population. Rapid weight loss after MBS may increase risk of refeeding syndrome, especially in the setting of receiving nutrition support therapy.[15]

Patients at risk for refeeding syndrome should receive 100 mg thiamin for at least the first 5 to 7 days of EN or PN.[15] Patients receiving EN can receive enteral repletion, and patients receiving PN should receive intravenous (IV) repletion. Providing thiamin to these patients ensures that thiamin requirements for carbohydrate metabolism are met. Patients require multivitamin supplementation as well. Patients requiring PN require daily IV multivitamins added to the PN. Patients receiving EN should receive enteral multivitamin supplementation for at least the first 10 days of therapy, but longer supplementation may be necessary. Readers are encouraged to review the ASPEN consensus paper for a comprehensive review of the refeeding syndrome.[15]

Nutrition Diagnosis

Box 8.7 lists nutrition diagnoses that may be made for MBS patients requiring nutrition support therapy.[5]

Nutrition Intervention

Enteral Nutrition

Enteral Access

For any patient requiring enteral access after MBS, determining the optimal route of access requires careful evaluation with the patient's surgeon.[16,17] Obtaining enteral access in patients after MBS can be a challenge given the altered GI anatomy, particularly for Roux-en-Y gastric bypass (RYGB) patients.

Short-term enteral access with a nasoenteric tube may require direct visualization for appropriate insertion. An RYGB patient scheduled for a planned surgical intervention may have a feeding tube inserted in the remnant stomach, or a feeding jejunostomy may be considered. At the time of this publication, there have been no case reports of enteral access in patients who have had sleeve gastrectomy. This author has seen a percutaneous endoscopic gastrostomy (PEG) inserted into a sleeve gastrectomy patient who developed dysphagia and progressed to end-stage kidney disease requiring hemodialysis. The patient was able to tolerate EN with a concentrated formula designed for the dialysis patient population. The patient was eventually able to take a small amount of a texture-modified diet and was able to transition to a night-cycled EN

BOX 8.7 Selected Nutrition Diagnoses for Metabolic and Bariatric Surgery Patients Requiring Nutrition Support[6]

Increased energy expenditure
Inadequate energy intake
Predicted suboptimal energy intake
Inadequate oral intake
Inadequate fluid intake
Increased nutrient needs
Inadequate protein-energy intake
Inadequate protein intake
Inadequate vitamin intake (specify)
Inadequate mineral intake (specify)
Swallowing difficulty
Altered gastrointestinal function
Unintended weight loss
Malnutrition

schedule. More case reports are necessary to determine the optimal enteral access devices for patients who have had sleeve gastrectomy.

The RDN has an important role in advocating for the appropriate enteral access device for MBS patients requiring EN. This is particularly important when the primary team taking care of the patient is not the MBS team. When the discussion of enteral access arises, the RDN can remind the team of the patient's unique anatomy and advocate for the best feeding tube and access site based on the patient's surgical history.

Formula Selection

The selection of enteral formula depends on the patient's energy, protein, and fluid requirements as well as the underlying condition and comorbidities.[1,17]

- For patients with otherwise normal digestive and absorptive capacity, a standard polymeric enteral formula should be sufficient.

- A fiber-containing enteral formula may be beneficial for patients who require long-term enteral support or for those with diarrhea or constipation.
- Patients requiring a volume restriction (eg, patients with heart failure) benefit from a concentrated enteral formula to limit fluid delivery. Concentrated enteral formulas often contain some sucrose and may lead to dumping syndrome if infused rapidly into the gastric pouch. Controlled feeding with an enteral feeding pump should help avoid this problem.
- Patients with kidney failure may require a concentrated enteral formula restricted in sodium, potassium, and phosphorus.

A comprehensive review of enteral formula selection is beyond the scope of this chapter; detailed information is available in Roberts and colleagues.[17]

Type of Infusion

The type of infusion primarily depends on the location of the feeding tube, as follows[1]:

- Patients being fed into the remnant stomach could receive bolus feedings. Bolus feedings are typically between 250 and 500 mL and are infused rapidly into the stomach.
- Patients being fed into the gastric pouch, into the gastric sleeve, or into the small intestine cannot tolerate bolus feedings because the gastric pouch, sleeve, and small intestine do not have the appropriate reservoir capacity. These patients require pump-assisted enteral feedings, starting with continuous infusion and transitioning to a cycled regimen if they are discharged on EN. There are no evidence-based guidelines for the maximum enteral feeding rate for pump-assisted feedings, so the rate is best determined by patient tolerance.

Micronutrient Supplementation

Most enteral formulas meet 100% of the Dietary Reference Intakes for most vitamins and minerals.[17] However, to prevent deficiencies, MBS patients requiring EN should receive the same amounts of vitamin and mineral supplementation as MBS patients on an oral diet. In addition, any known micronutrient deficiency should be corrected following the standard repletion guidelines for patients on an oral diet. See Appendix C for supplementation recommendations and Appendix D for information on the repletion of micronutrient deficiencies.

Parenteral Nutrition

Parenteral Access

PN patients require dedicated central venous access as follows[18]:

- For short-term PN (less than 6 to 8 weeks), a peripherally inserted central catheter is an appropriate choice for access.
- For long-term PN (typically longer than 8 weeks), a tunneled central venous access device is the most appropriate choice.

Initiating and Advancing Parenteral Nutrition

To avoid worsening electrolyte abnormalities and hyperglycemia, the patient should have normal serum electrolytes and blood glucose before PN is initiated. PN should be initiated with a low dextrose concentration (150 to 200 g or lessdextrose in the first 24 hours) and advanced progressively to the goals for volume, dextrose, amino acids, and fat emulsion over the next 2 to 3 days. Refer to Roberts and Kirsch[17] or your facility clinician for information on calculating the PN solution.

For the first 3 to 5 days of PN, potassium, phosphorus, and magnesium should be monitored at least daily to assess for refeeding syndrome. PN advancement should be delayed if the patient shows signs of refeeding syndrome.[18]

Administration of Micronutrients

Patients receiving PN should be provided IV vitamins and trace elements daily (see Boxes 8.8 and 8.9 on page 196).[18] In general, these micronutrients can be provided in standard amounts because IV infusion eliminates the risk of malabsorption. If micronutrient deficiencies are identified, IV or intramuscular repletion should be provided when possible.

BOX 8.8 Daily Parenteral Vitamin Requirements[18]

Vitamin A	1 mg (3,300 IU)
Vitamin D	5 mcg (200 IU)
Vitamin E	10 mg (10 IU)
Vitamin K	150 mcg
Vitamin C	200 mg
Biotin	60 mcg
Vitamin B12	5 mcg
Folic acid	600 mcg
Niacin	40 mg
Pantothenic acid	15 mg
Pyridoxine	6 mg
Riboflavin	3.6 mg

BOX 8.9 Daily Parenteral Trace Element Requirements[18]

Chromium	10 to 15 mcg
Copper	0.3 to 0.5 mg
Manganese	60 to 100 mcg or based on serum levels
Selenium	20 to 60 mcg
Zinc	2.5 to 5 mg

Monitoring and Evaluation

Enteral Nutrition Patients

Box 8.10 on pages 198 to 199 identifies typical complications associated with EN and possible intervention strategies.[16] Electrolytes, including magnesium and phosphorus, should be monitored daily for at least the first 3 to 5 days of EN, particularly if the patient is at risk for refeeding syndrome or has excessive electrolyte losses (eg, from diarrhea or high-output fistula). Once the patient is stable, monitoring can be done less frequently.[16,19]

Parenteral Nutrition Patients

PN patients should be monitored for metabolic complications. Electrolyte levels (including magnesium and phosphorus) should be assessed daily. Blood glucose levels should be closely monitored because of the increased risk of hyperglycemia in this population.

PN patients also need to be monitored for complications associated with central venous access, including infections and mechanical problems with the central venous access device.[18]

The patient's hydration status and weight should be monitored regularly. Box 8.11 on pages 200 to 201 identifies typical complications associated with PN and possible intervention strategies.[16]

Changing Route of Administration

As the patient's clinical status improves, they may be able to transition from PN to EN, from PN to an oral diet, or from EN to an oral diet. The RDN should follow the patient's status closely and advocate for transitioning as appropriate. During transition times, the risk for under- or overfeeding increases, and intensive monitoring is crucial to prevent these complications.

BOX 8.10 Management Strategies for Enteral Nutrition Complications[16]

Abdominal pain/bloating

Assess for constipation.

Decrease flow rate of infusion.

If bolus feeding, change to continuous infusion.

Avoid use of liquid medications containing sugar alcohols.

Aspiration

Elevate head of bed more than 30° (preferably more than 45°) during infusion.

Do not bolus feed patients at high risk for aspiration.

Consider postpyloric feeding.

Constipation

Try fiber-containing formula.

Provide adequate fluid.

Initiate bowel regimen.

Dehydration

Monitor for early signs/symptoms.

Provide adequate water flushes.

Use standard dilution (ie, 1 kcal/mL) enteral formula.

Diarrhea

Check for infectious causes (eg, *Clostridium difficile*).

Use sterile technique when preparing formula for administration.

Review medication list—avoid elixirs, known cathartics.

Try fiber-containing formula.

Check osmolarity of formula—switch to isotonic formula if necessary.

Add antidiarrheal medications.

Consider use of probiotics.

Avoid use of liquid medications containing sugar alcohols.

BOX 8.10 Management Strategies for Enteral Nutrition Complications[16] (cont.)

Electrolyte disturbances

Monitor daily while initiating feedings; correct imbalances promptly.

Monitor long-term enteral patients every 1 to 3 months.

Feeding tube clog

Flush tube with 30 mL or more water every 4 hours.

Flush tube with 30 mL or more water before and after medication administration.

Use liquid forms of medication when possible.

Do not flush tube with cola or juices—these will coagulate proteins, worsening the clog.

Use a solution of pancreatic enzymes plus sodium bicarbonate or a commercial declogging device to address tube clogs.

Hyperglycemia

Avoid excessive energy delivery.

Consider fiber-containing formula.

Consider diabetes-specific formula.

Provide insulin as needed.

Infection around tube insertion site

Ensure meticulous tube care.

Refer patient to physician—may need antibiotics or antifungals.

Vitamin or mineral deficiency

Ensure that formula meets 100% of daily recommended intake.

Provide multivitamin/mineral elixir.

Provide separate vitamin or mineral supplementation if needed.

BOX 8.11 Management Strategies for Parenteral Nutrition Complications[16]

Catheter-related bloodstream infection

Use aseptic technique for insertion and catheter care.

Use aseptic technique when preparing parenteral nutrition (PN) for infusion.

Dedicate one port for PN infusion only.

Dehydration

Assess fluid requirements carefully.

Account for all fluid losses (eg, diarrhea, fistula output).

Monitor daily weight and input/output.

Provide supplemental intravenous (IV) fluid separately from PN if necessary.

Electrolyte disturbances

Monitor daily while initiating PN; consider twice per day laboratory testing for patients at high risk for refeeding syndrome.

Correct electrolyte abnormalities promptly.

Once electrolyte levels are stable, frequency of monitoring can be decreased.

Essential fatty acid deficiency

Provide adequate IV fat emulsion to meet essential fatty acid needs.

Monitor fatty acid profile, including triene-to-tetraene ratio, every 6 months.

Intestinal atrophy

Transition to EN as soon as possible.

For long-term PN patients, allow small amounts of oral nutrition, if possible.

Hyperglycemia

Give 150 to 200 g or less dextrose on the first day.

If blood glucose (BG) is higher than 180 mg/dL, check finger stick blood glucose (FSBG) every 6 hours and administer regular insulin.

Do not advance dextrose concentration until BG is within target range.

Add regular insulin directly to PN based on prior day's requirements (typically give two-thirds of prior day's requirements).

For cycled PN, check midcycle FSBG.

BOX 8.11 Management Strategies for Parenteral Nutrition Complications[16] (cont.)

Hypoglycemia

Follow BG trends carefully and decrease insulin if necessary.

For ambulatory, non–intensive care unit patients, goal BG is less than 180 mg/dL; stringent BG goal may lead to hypoglycemia.

For cycled PN, decrease infusion rate by one half before discontinuing PN.

Check FSBG 1 hour after PN is discontinued.

Metabolic bone disease

Provide adequate calcium and vitamin D.

Monitor bone density yearly.

Initiate appropriate therapy as indicated.

Parenteral nutrition-associated liver disease

Avoid overfeeding.

Avoid excessive fat delivery.

Cycle PN.

Volume overload

Assess fluid requirements carefully.

Review medical history for conditions requiring fluid restriction.

Concentrate PN solution as needed.

Treat with diuretics as indicated.

Vitamin or trace element deficiencies or excess

Provide vitamins and trace elements daily in PN.

Monitor vitamin and trace element panel every 6 months.

Replete individual vitamins and trace elements as indicated, either via PN, separate infusion, or orally (if that is the only available route).

High levels are most often seen with trace elements; if any levels are high, remove the commercial preparation and add back individual trace elements.

Team Approach

Management of the patient requiring nutrition support therapy after MBSrequires a team approach, as shown here:

- Before EN is initiated, the surgeon must be consulted to determine feasibility of EN and the best route for enteral access.
- Once EN is started, the RDN must work closely with the patient's nurse and physician to evaluate and manage complications.
- A pharmacist who has expertise in nutrition support can assist with electrolyte management and management of medications that can be added to the PN solution.

Multidisciplinary collaboration optimizes patient care, provides appropriate nutrition support therapy, and may minimize complications.

References

1. Boullata JI, Carrera AL, Harvey L, et al. ASPEN Safe practices for enteral nutrition therapy. *JPEN J Parenter Enteral Nutr.* 2017;41:15-103. doi:10.1177/0148607116673053
2. Worthington P, Balint J, Bechtold M, et al. When is parenteral nutrition appropriate? *JPEN J Parenter Enteral Nutr.* 2017;41:324-377. doi:10.1177/0148607117695251
3. Mechanick JI, Apovian C, Brethauer S, et al. Clinical practice guidelines for the perioperative nutritional, metabolic, and nonsurgical support of patients undergoing bariatric procedures—2019 update: cosponsored by American Association of Clinical Endocrinologists/American College of Endocrinology, the Obesity Society, American Society for Metabolic and Bariatric Surgery, Obesity Medicine Association and American Societ of Anesthesiologists. *Obesity.* 2020;28:O1-O58.
4. Kumpf VJ, Slocum K, Binkley J, Jensen G. Complications after bariatric surgery: survey evaluating impact on the practice of specialized nutrition support. *Nutr Clin Pract.* 2007;22:673-678. doi:10.1177/0115426507022006673

5. Clave SA, Taylor BE, Martindale RG, et al. Guidelines for the provision and assessment of nutrition support therapy in the adult critically ill patient: Society of Critical Care Medicine (SCCM) and American Society for Parenteral and Enteral Nutrition (A.S.P.E.N.). *JPEN J Parenter Enteral Nutr.* 2016;40:159-211. doi:10.1177/0148607115621863
6. Academy of Nutrition and Dietetics. *eNCPT: Nutrition Care Process Terminology* (online publication). Academy of Nutrition and Dietetics; 2019.
7. Chen Y. Acute bariatric surgery complications: managing parenteral nutrition in the morbidly obese. *J Am Diet Assoc.* 2010;110:1734-1737. doi:10.1016/j.jada.2010.08.010
8. Mogensen KM, Andrew BY, Corona JC, Robinson MK. Validation of the Society for Critical Care Medicine and American Society for Parenteral and Enteral Nutrition recommendatios for caloric provision to critically ill obese patients: a pilot study. *JPEN J Parenter Enteral Nutr.* 2016;40:713-721. doi:10.1177/0148607115584001
9. Academy of Nutrition and Dietetics Evidence Analysis Library. Critical illness evidence-based nutrition practice guideline 2012. Accessed May 5, 2014. http://andevidencelibrary.com/topic.cfm?cat=4800
10. Berge JE, Goon A, Choban PS, Flancbaum L. Efficacy of hypocaloric TPN in hospitalized obese patients: a prospective, double-blind randomized trial. *JPEN J Parenter Enteral Nutr.* 1994;18:203-207. doi:10.1177/0148607194018003203
11. Choban PS, Burg JC, Scales D, Flancbaum L. Hypo-energetic nutrition support in hospitalized obese patients. *Am J Clin Nutr.* 1997;66:546-550.
12. Choban P, Dickerson R, Malone A, Worthington P, Compher C. A.S.P.E.N. clinical guidelines: nutrition support of hospitalized adult patients with obesity. *JPEN J Parenter Enteral Nutr.* 2013;37:714-744. doi:10.1177/0148607113499374
13. Canada TW, Lord LM. Fluids, electrolytes, and acid-based disorders. In: Mueller CM, Lord LM, Marian M, McClave SA, Miller SJ, eds. *The ASPEN Nutrition Support Core Curriculum.* 3rd ed. American Society for Enteral and Parenteral Nutrition; 2017:113-137.
14. Becker DA, Balcer LJ, Galetta SL. The neurological complications of nutritional deficiency following bariatric surgery. *J Obesity.* 2012;2012:608534. doi:10.1155/2012/608534
15. da Silva JSV, Seres DS, Sabino K, et al. ASPEN consensus recommendations for refeeding syndrome. *Nutr Clin Pract.* 2020;35:178-195. doi:10.1002/ncp.10474
16. Mogensen KM. Nutrition support therapy for the bariatric surgery patient. *Weight Manage Matters.* 2010;7:8-16.

17. Roberts S, Kirsch R. Enteral nutrition formulations. In: Mueller CM, Lord LM, Marian M, McClave SA, Miller SJ, eds. *The ASPEN Nutrition Support Core Curriculum*. 3rd ed. American Society for Parenteral and Enteral Nutrition; 2017:227-249.
18. Mirtallo J, Canada T, Johnson D, et al. Safe practices for parenteral nutrition. *JPEN J Parenter Enteral Nutr.* 2004;28(suppl):S39-S70. doi:10.1177/0148607104028006s39
19. Doley J, Phillips W. Overview of enteral nutrition. In: Mueller CM, Lord LM, Marian M, McClave SA, Miller SJ, eds. *The ASPEN Nutrition Support Core Curriculum*. 3rd ed. American Society for Parenteral and Enteral Nutrition; 2017:213-225.

CHAPTER 9

Endoscopic Bariatric Therapies

Introduction

Endoscopic bariatric therapies (EBTs) have continued to gain popularity in the United States and abroad as more Food and Drug Administration (FDA)-approved devices hit the market. This can be attributed to the fact that there has been a significant gap between the prevalence of obesity in the international populace and the utilization of the available obesity treatments. Although metabolic and bariatric surgery (MBS) is known to be an efficacious treatment for weight loss, less than 1% of qualified patients move forward with surgery due to access to care, fear of surgical risks, as well as financial burden.[1] Meanwhile, standard lifestyle interventions even with the addition of weight loss medications typically result in only a 3% to 10% total body weight loss.[2] This leaves many patients facing the tough decision between minimal weight loss and permanent anatomic changes. EBTs provide an option that offers a moderate weight loss with minimal invasiveness and are typically approved for a lower body mass index (BMI). In addition, EBTs can serve as a bridge therapy to provide short-term, nonpermanent weight loss intended to help patients qualify for surgeries, such as bariatric surgeries, organ transplants, or joint replacements. Due to the nonpermanent nature of many of these therapies, they often do not exclude patients from getting bariatric surgery at a later point. The nascent development and marketing of these devices and procedures renders little evidence or literature to guide the nutritional care provided to these patients. The intention of this chapter is to elucidate nutritional guidelines for each device/procedure based on protocols used in large clinical trials, as well as what is typically seen in general practice.

Intragastric Balloons

Mechanism of Action

Intragastric balloons (IGBs) help patients lose weight by lowering preprandial hunger and increasing postprandial satiety.[3] From preliminary research, experts hypothesize that this effect is achieved by the balloons acting on gastro mechanoreceptors to stimulate vagal signaling to brain regions associated with hunger, as well as delaying gastric emptying and taking up space in the stomach.[4,5] It is interesting to note that age, baseline BMI, and the degree of delay of gastric emptying are all associated with the amount of weight loss seen. Evidence shows that female patients[‡] aged 40 years old or less lose more weight than older female patients.[6,7] For fluid-filled balloons, lower baseline BMI results in greater excess weight loss (EWL), and greater increase in gastric retention is associated with more weight loss.[6,7] There are currently two IGBs that are FDA approved and being used in clinical practice: a single fluid-filled balloon system and a three gas-filled balloon system.

Single Fluid-Filled Balloon System

The single fluid-filled balloon system is the most common IGB and received FDA approval in August 2015.[7] Recent data from a registry study of clinical patients showed 11.8 ±7.5% total body weight loss (TBWL) at 6 months.[8] This balloon is placed endoscopically and filled with saline between 400 and 700 mL. It has a residence time of 6 months, at which point the patient will undergo a repeat endoscopy to puncture, deflate, and remove the balloon through the patient's mouth.

‡ Data on sex assigned at birth or gender identity was not further specified, and specific recommendations or data for transgender and gender-diverse people were not provided. Please see pages xxi to xxii for more on gender-inclusive terminology.

Three Gas-Filled Balloons System

The swallowable gas-filled IGB is novel for the fact that it does not require an endoscopy to place the device, though it will still require a removal endoscopy. The patient swallows a capsule with a catheter attached, which fills the balloon to a volume of 250 mL with a nitrogen mix gas. Once filled, the catheter is detached and removed. This placement process is repeated for the second and third balloon at 2 weeks and 8 weeks from the initial placement procedure. Like the fluid-filled balloon, the gas-filled balloons have a 6-month residence time at which point an endoscopy is required to puncture and remove all three balloons. A recent analysis of clinical patients showed a weight loss of 9.9 ±6.2% TBWL at the 6-month removal time point.[9]

Intragastric Balloon Nutritional Recommendations

As is common with all EBTs, there is little research on the most effective way to provide nutritional counseling to IGB patients. While that is true, we can learn from the lifestyle programs designed for the pivotal trials of these devices. The large clinical trials of the IGBs used a moderate-intensity lifestyle therapy program in accordance with the 2013 American Heart Association/American College of Cardiology/The Obesity Society Guidelines for management of overweight and obesity in adults, with a goal weight loss of 1.5 to 2 lb per week, meaning there were six to 13 sessions with a lifestyle therapy provider over the first 6 months.[10-12] It is best practice to see EBT patients with a frequency at least matching the moderate-intensity lifestyle with a nutrition counseling session once a month and the opportunity to attend support groups.[13] The nutrition follow-up should continue for a full year after placement, which includes the 6 months after the balloon is removed in order to help combat weight regain. The exact nutrition counseling program will vary based on the provider's practice, but it typically includes a reduced-calorie diet with a 500 to 1,000 kcal reduction from basal metabolic rate to promote a 1- to 2-lb weight loss per week. Exercise prescription should be in line with the

Physical Activity Guidelines for Americans, second edition, which encourages 150 to 300 minutes a week of moderate intensity or 75 to 150 minutes a week of vigorous-intensity aerobic physical activity.[14] The nutrition counseling should employ education and counseling techniques, such as those listed in Appendix H, and should be reflective of the Academy of Nutrition and Dietetics position on counseling patients for weight loss.[15]

Although the long-term nutrition counseling for IGB patients should not differ much from a typical weight loss diet, two aspects that require some unique handling are the preprocedure and postprocedure diets and the nutritional treatment of accommodative symptoms. Prior to balloon placement, patients should have no food or drink starting at midnight, with only small sips of water to take medications. After device placement for the gas-filled balloons, patients should be on a clear liquid diet and advance to a full liquid diet over the course of 24 hours as tolerated. After 24 hours if the patient is feeling well, they can expand their diet back to a regular solid food, calorie-reduced, weight loss diet. A barrier that a registered dietitian nutritionist (RDN) should anticipate is that there is limited insurance coverage for these procedures. It is likely that patients will be self-pay, adding a challenge to getting patients to return for follow-up unless the program is structured as pay in advance.

For the fluid-filled balloons, the accommodative symptoms can be more severe than gas-filled balloons. It is important to stay in contact with patients, and, if symptoms are persistent, the patient may need to return to clinic for intravenous (IV) fluids. Patients will need to stay on a clear liquid diet for the first 72 hours, after which they can advance to full liquids for 1 day, then a pureed diet until 10 days post placement. If a patient is doing very well at the 1-week follow-up visit, they may advance at day 7 through 9 and should be on a reduced-calorie soft diet, and finally after day 9 they will return to a reduced-calorie solid-food diet. For both the gas- and fluid-filled balloons, experts recommended that patients avoid gastric irritants (eg, alcohol, carbonation, caffeine) while on an altered consistency diet. The biggest nutritional concerns immediately after placement are maintaining hydration especially if the patient experiences vomiting, and maintaining a protein level around 60 g per day. To navigate these potential hurdles, practitioners should tell patients to sip water through the day with a goal of 64 fluid ounces. Sports drinks with electrolytes (eg, Pedialyte) should be kept on hand in case of vomiting or difficulty consuming adequate fluids. When tolerated, patients are recommended to incorporate one to two protein shakes or flavorless protein power (eg, Beneprotein) in broths/soups into their daily intake. Symptom severity can fluctuate widely between patients, and it is important that they have a contact number to reach out to in the situation that they are feeling unwell.

Symptoms commonly seen with the balloons include persistent nausea, vomiting, generalized abdominal pain or discomfort, back pain, and reflux.[4] Most of these can be managed with medical therapy and altered consistency diets. Symptoms that are present approximately 1 month after placement are more chronic issues. In practice, one of the most common chronic symptoms with gas-filled balloons is a persistent gnawing sensation in the stomach that resolves after eating a small amount of food. To help treat this, it is best to advise patients to consume a full glass of cold water, try real peppermint (eg, Altoids or peppermint tea), or eat a small snack (less than 50 kcal). If this does not resolve symptoms or the need for consistent snacking to treat symptoms is sabotaging weight loss, then it is best to escalate the issue to the treating physician for medical management.

Another common chronic symptom group includes bloating, gas, constipation, and occasionally vomiting. Based on observation, this occurs most frequently with a sudden increase in fiber intake or a high-fat meal. The thought is that these difficult to digest nutrients may be further slowing the already delayed gastric emptying, resulting in this uncomfortable group of symptoms. One suggested treatment is to reduce fiber intake to 10 to 12 g per day and avoid high-fat meals, such as those containing fried foods. This decrease in fiber unfortunately will limit the patient's intake of many healthy fiber-rich foods, so it is essential to work with them to focus on calorie reduction and finding ways to incorporate low-calorie healthy options. Another possible source of symptoms is delayed gastric emptying, which can necessitate a short course of liquid diet (3 to 7 days) and a prokinetic agent like erythromycin or metoclopramide (Reglan). The symptoms typically associated with delayed gastric emptying include vomiting, bloating, or fetid eructation. If abdominal pain worsens, refer back to the physician due to risk of hyperinflation, pancreatitis, or gastric perforation. This symptom management is a great place for the RDN to shine as a source of support for the IGB patients.

Aspiration Therapy

Aspiration therapy received FDA approval in June 2016 for patients with a BMI of 35 to 55. It involves placing a gastrostomy tube, which attaches to a secondary device, to allow patients to aspirate gastric contents approximately 20 minutes after a meal.[7] Patients use a reservoir to deliver clean water into the stomach, which then mixes with gastric contents and drains out for disposal, thus removing approximately 30% of calories prior to reaching the intestines for further absorption.[7,16] Aspiration therapy patients showed a 1-year weight loss of 14.2% to 21.5% TBWL and were able to maintain this weight loss if therapy continued for another year. There is no current limitation for how long the aspiration tube may remain in place, which offers a long-term therapy, unlike some of the alternative EBT options. Data published for patients who have undergone 4 years of aspiration therapy show continued improvement in markers of cardiometabolic health and quality of life. There is also no evidence of development of abnormal eating behavior based on comprehensive psychological interview assessments. Bomb calorimetry studies of the aspirate demonstrate that a patient's weight loss cannot be solely attributed to calories aspirated.[17] The rest of the weight loss is due to new healthy lifestyle behaviors, which the RDN can support, such as making healthier food choices, eating slower, chewing more, and increasing water intake.

Aspiration Therapy Nutritional Recommendations

Similar to IGB, the intensity and focus of the nutrition therapy will vary based on the physician's practice, patients are advised to follow a moderate-intensity lifestyle therapy program in accordance with the American Heart Association/American College of Cardiology/The Obesity Society 2013 guidelines for management of overweight and obesity in adults.[12] There is little available in the way of evidence-based recommendations, but in practice, there is a typical postprocedure diet progression. This starts with no food or drinks at midnight before device placement except for small sips of water to take medication. After device placement only clear liquids are allowed for the first 24 hours. After 24 hours, patients can begin to gradually expand to their regular reduced-calorie diet as tolerated. They can start tracking food intake and practice chewing foods well. The patient should return to the clinic 2 weeks after device placement to be trained on how to start aspiration therapy and placement of skin port. Once training is complete the patient should remain on a pureed diet for 1 week, followed by a soft/ground diet for 1 week. This allows for a learning curve in aspiration without experiencing clogs in the tubing. At 1 month after device placement, the patient will be able to return to a regular reduced-calorie diet with an energy prescription based on an energy equation adjusted for a 1- to 2-lb weight loss per week. This energy prescription, in addition to aspiration therapy, allows for the potential for faster weight loss or for some deviations from diet while maintaining a healthy weight loss rate.

Once patients are on their reduced-calorie diet, there are several important aspects to success with aspiration therapy. Primarily, all foods must be chewed to an applesauce-like consistency. A good rule is to chew 25 times or more per bite prior to swallowing to avoid tube clogs. With each meal patients should drink at least 8 fl oz ounces of water to assist with flow of the aspirate. Even with increased mastication, there are some foods that are difficult to aspirate, per patient reports. This can vary from patient to patient and may take some individual experimentation to develop an understanding of what can be aspirated vs what needs to be avoided or not aspirated. Some commonly reported difficult foods are steak, nuts, seeds, hot dogs, and fibrous vegetables. Ideally each patient would aspirate two to three times per day, 20 minutes after meals that are greater than 250 kcal, and each aspiration will be around 10 to 20 minutes. Many RDNs worry about nutrition deficiencies in these patients; however, no clinically significant metabolic or electrolyte disorders were observed in the 4-year data from the 10-center randomized controlled trial.[18] Mild hypokalemia was only seen in four patients across all study sites, and this was successfully treated with potassium supplementation.[16] Taking an over-the-counter multivitamin is recommended as a precaution due to the reduced-calorie nature of the diet. This is a device that requires a significant time and lifestyle commitment, and it is important to find patients who are ready for this change. If properly utilized, it has the potential to result in significant weight loss.

Endoscopic Sleeve Gastroplasty

The endoscopic sleeve gastroplasty (ESG) is a procedure that uses an FDA-approved suturing device to reduce the gastric volume to mimic the surgical sleeve; however, it is done endoscopically and results in minimal permanent anatomical changes caused by scar formation.[19] The sutures transform the shape of the stomach into a tube-like form that reduces stomach volume by up to 70%. This helps to decrease preprandial hunger, increase postprandial satiety, and increase feeling of fullness.[20] In addition to the obvious increase in fullness from reduction in stomach volume, the ESG is also associated with delayed gastric emptying and an improved metabolic profile in patients with obesity.[21] Data from a recently published meta-analysis of 1,772 patients showed 15.1% TBWL at 6 months, 16.5% at 12 months, and 17.2% at 18 to 24 months.[22]

As with other EBTs, patients who followed up most frequently with a nutritional and psychological team member experienced the greatest weight loss success.[23] The best practice is meeting with a nutrition, psychological, and exercise professional every 1 to 2 weeks. There are limited medical centers performing this procedure, which requires many patients to travel long distances and creates a barrier to frequent nutrition follow-up visits. This creates an opportunity for the RDN to advocate telehealth in order to encourage follow-up compliance. The literature on ESG patients suggests the following diet progression: a liquid diet starting the day before the procedure up to 2 weeks after the procedure, then an altered consistency diet of pureed then soft/ground foods progressing as tolerated over the course of 4 to 6 weeks.[24] After the diet progression is complete, the patient should be able to follow a regular reduced-calorie diet with a reduction in calorie prescription to create a 1- to 2-lb weight loss per week. The nutrition follow-up should continue for a full year in order to establish permanent healthy habits and prevent weight loss regain.[20] One of the unique nutritional concerns seen in practice is maintenance of protein levels around 60 to 80 g to help with satiation and healing postprocedure. During this time, patients often depend on protein drinks and should be advised on the best low-sugar and low-calorie options. Since there is significant restriction immediately postprocedure, it is best to warn patients that it may be hard to maintain hydration, so it is best to consistently sip water throughout the day and not drink large volumes during meals. In order to prevent an uncomfortable sensation of fullness or possibly an episode of emesis, patients should eat small amounts several times a day, set utensils down between bites, chew well, and stop eating at the beginning signs of fullness. With the help of an RDN and these healthy lifestyle changes, the ESG can be an effective minimally invasive tool to help patients who are averse to permanent anatomic changes or have a BMI too low for surgery.

Revision Procedures

Revisional procedures are intended to endoscopically treat weight regain after surgical procedures. The causes of the weight regain range from returning to unhealthy lifestyle habits, psychological barriers including substance abuse, as well as anatomical shifts from the surgical alteration.[25] One anatomical change that has garnered a lot of attention is a dilation in the gastrojejunal anastomosis, which results in a loss in the sensation of early satiety that causes much of the weight loss associated with the Roux-en-Y gastric bypass.[26,27] The transoral outlet reduction procedure requires the endoscopist to measure the stoma, use argon plasma coagulation to create scarring around the stoma, then deploy a suturing device to sew down the anastomosis until the stoma is only 4 to 8 mm in diameter.[28] This endoscopic revision of the stoma has been demonstrated to stop weight regain in 77% to 100% of the postbariatric patient population and results in a 12-month weight loss ranging from 5.83 ± 11 kg to 10.5± 12.5 kg.[29] It is recommended that patients are nothing by mouth (NPO) the night before the procedure, start a clear liquid diet for 3 days postprocedure, advance to a full liquid diet from day 3 to 7, follow a pureed then soft diet over the course of 4 weeks, and at 6 weeks postprocedure return to their regular reduced-calorie diet.[28] Although there is little to suggest what kind of nutrition therapy program is best for these patients, it is advisable that they receive some follow-up support to prevent weight regain. Ensuring that these patients have nutritional follow-up care is essential to their success and can be limited if the patient is seeing a physician who is not part of a bariatric practice. It is important for RDNs to advocate to patients that they seek out a physician who has a nutrition follow-up program in place. There is also an increased need for protein in these patients, and, in practice, it is recommended that a patient reach a goal of 80 g protein per day or return to their postoperative protein recommendation, whichever is the higher amount.

Emerging Therapies

EBTs are an exciting and quickly evolving field with many new therapies still in various stages of receiving FDA approval in order to be brought to market. There are several on the radar that each offers unique contributions in the progression of the technology. There is a single swallowable fluid-filled balloon that deflates and passes out of the gastrointestinal tract on its own, thereby eliminating the need for an endoscopy.[7] Another procedure is an endoscopically placed and removed saline-filled balloon that can remain in place for 9 months rather than the standard 6 months and has an inflation tube that allows for volume adjustments while in residence.[7,30] The primary obesity surgery endoluminal (POSE) procedure is another suturing procedure currently under FDA review that reduces gastric volume.[30] The transpyloric shuttle is an additional device that spans the pylorus with two bulb connected by a tether, whose mechanism of action is to cause intermittent gastric obstruction.[7] The incisionless anastomosis system operates by using two endoscopically placed magnets that find each other in the intestines and create an anastomosis, thereby bypassing a large portion of the intestine.[7] This system allows for bidirectional flow through the native pathway and the new anastomosis. Without a doubt in this ever-evolving field, new and innovative therapies will continue to emerge and impact the medical landscape.

Conclusion

The development of EBTs expands the treatable population, hopefully decreasing the burden of obesity-related diseases on our health care system. RDNs play an essential role in the treatment by evaluating patients for candidacy for providing nutrition and calorie prescriptions, for the first line of symptom management, for providing support, and as communication links between physician and patient. Hopefully as this field continues to develop and RDNs see more patients, there will be an increase in evidence-based guidelines and a clearer view of best treatment practices. In the fight against the obesity epidemic, it is essential that medical professionals be aware of all the tools available to properly support and treat this growing patient population.

References

1. Ponce J, DeMaria EJ, Nguyen NT, et al. American Society for Metabolic and Bariatric Surgery estimation of bariatric surgery procedures in 2015 and surgeon workforce in the United States. *Surg Obes Relat Dis.* 2016;12(9):1637-1639.
2. Khera R, Murad MH, Chandar AK, et al. Association of pharmacological treatments for obesity with weight loss and adverse events: a systematic review and meta-analysis [published correction appears in *JAMA*. 2016 Sep 6;316(9):995]. *JAMA.* 2016;315(22):2424-2434. doi:10.1001/jama.2016.7602
3. Ribeiro da Silva J, Proença L, Rodrigues A, et al. Intragastric balloon for obesity treatment: safety, tolerance, and efficacy. *GE Port J Gastroenterol.* 2018;25(5):236-242. doi:10.1159/000485428
4. Tate CM, Geliebter A. Intragastric balloon treatment for obesity: review of recent studies. *Adv Ther.* 2017;34(8):1859-1875. doi:10.1007/s12325-017-0562-3
5. Gómez V, Woodman G, Abu Dayyeh BK. Delayed gastric emptying as a proposed mechanism of action during intragastric balloon therapy: results of a prospective study. *Obesity (Silver Spring).* 2016;24(9):1849-1853. doi:10.1002/oby.215556
6. Diab AF, Abdurasul EM, Diab FH. The effect of age, gender, and baseline BMI on weight loss outcomes in obese patients undergoing intragastric balloon therapy. *Obes Surg.* 2019;29(11):3542-3546. doi:10.1007/s11695-019-04023-y

7. Shahnazarian V, Ramai D, Sarkar A. Endoscopic bariatric therapies for treating obesity: a learning curve for gastroenterologists. *Transl Gastroenterol Hepatol*. 2019;4:16. doi:10.21037/tgh.2019.03.01
8. Vargas EJ, Pesta CM, Bali A, et al. Single fluid-filled intragastric balloon safe and effective for inducing weight loss in a real-world population. *Clin Gastroenterol Hepatol*. 2018;16(7):1073-1080.e1. doi:10.1016/j.cgh.2018.01.046
9. Moore RL, Seger MV, Garber SM, et al. Clinical safety and effectiveness of a swallowable gas-filled intragastric balloon system for weight loss: consecutively treated patients in the initial year of U.S. commercialization. *Surg Obes Relat Dis*. 2019;15(3):417-423. doi:10.1016/j.soard.2018.12.007
10. Sullivan S, Swain J, Woodman G, et al. Randomized sham-controlled trial of the 6-month swallowable gas-filled intragastric balloon system for weight loss. *Surg Obes Relat Dis*. 2018;14(12):1876-1889. doi:10.1016/j.soard.2018.09.486
11. Ponce J, Woodman G, Swain J, et al. The REDUCE pivotal trial: a prospective, randomized controlled pivotal trial of a dual intragastric balloon for the treatment of obesity. *Surg Obes Relat Dis*. 2015;11(4):874-881. doi:10.1016/j.soard.2014.12.006
12. Apovian CM, Aronne LJ. The 2013 American Heart Association/American College of Cardiology/The Obesity Society Guideline for the Management of Overweight and Obesity in Adults. *Circulation*. 2015;132(16):1586-1591. doi:10.1161/circulationaha.114.010772
13. Sullivan S, Kumar N, Edmundowicz SA, et al. ASGE position statement on endoscopic bariatric therapies in clinical practice. *Gastrointestinal Endoscopy*. 2015;82(5):767-772. doi:10.1016/j.gie.2015.06.038
14. Piercy KL, Troiano RP, Ballard RM, et al. The physical activity guidelines for Americans. *JAMA*. 2018;320(19):2020-2028. doi:10.1001/jama.2018.14854
15. Raynor HA, Champagne CM. Position of the Academy of Nutrition and Dietetics: interventions for the treatment of overweight and obesity in adults. *J Acad Nutr Diet*. 2016;116(1):129-147. doi:10.1016/j.jand.2015.10.031
16. Thompson CC, Abu Dayyeh BK, Kushner R, et al. Percutaneous gastrostomy device for the treatment of Class II and Class III obesity: results of a randomized controlled trial. *Am J Gastroenterol*. 2017;112(3):447-457. doi:10.1038/ajg.2016.500
17. Sullivan S. Aspiration therapy for obesity. *Gastrointest Endosc Clin N Am*. 2017;27(2):277-288. doi:10.1016/j.giec.2016.12.001

18. Thompson CC, Abu Dayyeh BK, Kushnir V, et al. Aspiration therapy for the treatment of obesity: 4-year results of a multicenter randomized controlled trial. *Surg Obes Relat Dis*. 2019;15(8):1348-1354. doi:10.1016/j.soard.2019.04.026
19. Lopez-Nava G, Sharaiha RZ, Vargas EJ, et al. Endoscopic sleeve gastroplasty for obesity: a multicenter study of 248 patients with 24 months follow-up. *Obes Surg*. 2017;27(10):2649-2655. doi:10.1007/s11695-017-2693-7
20. Sartoretto A, Sui Z, Hill C, et al. Endoscopic Sleeve Gastroplasty (ESG) is a reproducible and effective endoscopic bariatric therapy suitable for widespread clinical adoption: a large, international multicenter study. *Obes Surg*. 2018;28(7):1812-1821. doi:10.1007/s11695-018-3135-x
21. Abu Dayyeh BK, Acosta A, Camilleri M, et al. Endoscopic Sleeve Gastroplasty alters gastric physiology and induces loss of body weight in obese individuals. *Clin Gastroenterol Hepatol*. 2017;15(1):37-43.e1. doi:10.1016/j.cgh.2015.12.030
22. Hedjoudje A, Abu Dayyeh BK, Cheskin LJ, et al. Efficacy and safety of endoscopic sleeve gastroplasty: a systematic review and meta-analysis. *Clin Gastroenterol Hepatol*. 2020;18(5):1043-1053.e4. doi:10.1016/j.cgh.2019.08.022
23. Lopez-Nava G, Galvao M, Bautista-Castaño I, Fernandez-Corbelle JP, Trell M. Endoscopic sleeve gastroplasty with 1-year follow-up: factors predictive of success. *Endosc Int Open*. 2016;4(2):E222-E227. doi:10.1055/s-0041-110771
24. Lopez-Nava G, Galvão MP, Bautista-Castaño I, Fernandez-Corbelle JP, Trell M, Lopez N. Endoscopic sleeve gastroplasty for obesity treatment: two years of experience. *Arq Bras Cir Dig*. 2017;30(1):18-20. doi:10.1590/0102-6720201700010006
25. Karmali S, Brar B, Shi X, Sharma AM, de Gara C, Birch DW. Weight recidivism post-bariatric surgery: a systematic review. *Obes Surg*. 2013;23(11):1922-1933. doi:10.1007/s11695-013-1070-4
26. Abu Dayyeh BK, Lautz DB, Thompson CC. Gastrojejunal stoma diameter predicts weight regain after Roux-en-Y gastric bypass. *Clin Gastroenterol Hepatol*. 2011;9(3):228-233. doi:10.1016/j.cgh.2010.11.004
27. Thompson CC, Chand B, Chen YK, et al. Endoscopic suturing for transoral outlet reduction increases weight loss after Roux-en-Y gastric bypass surgery. *Gastroenterology*. 2013;145(1):129-137.e3. doi:10.1053/j.gastro.2013.04.002
28. Hedberg HM, Trenk A, Kuchta K, Linn JG, Carbray J, Ujiki MB. Endoscopic gastrojejunostomy revision is more effective than medical management alone to address weight regain after RYGB. *Surg Endosc*. 2018;32(3):1564-1571. doi:10.1007/s00464-018-6073-8

29. Vargas EJ, Bazerbachi F, Rizk M, et al. Transoral outlet reduction with full thickness endoscopic suturing for weight regain after gastric bypass: a large multicenter international experience and meta-nalysis. *Surg Endosc.* 2018;32(1):252-259. doi:10.1007/s00464-017-5671-1

30. Bennett MC, Badillo R, Sullivan S. Endoscopic management [published correction appears in *Gastroenterol Clin North Am.* 2017 Jun;46(2):xvii]. *Gastroenterol Clin North Am.* 2016;45(4):673-688. doi:10.1016/j.gtc.2016.07.005

APPENDIX A

Online Resources

Academy of Nutrition and Dietetics

www.eatright.org
This site provides nutrition information on a variety of topics, such as hydration, food labels, and healthy mealtime eating, as well as a body mass index (BMI) calculator, reading lists, and recipes. There is also a feature for finding a dietitian using the "find an expert" tool.

Academy of Nutrition and Dietetics Evidence Analysis Library (EAL)

http://andevidencelibrary.com
The Nutrition Care in Bariatric Surgery section summarizes literature on postoperative medical nutrition therapy, postoperative energy needs, postoperative energy intake, postoperative macronutrient intake, weight loss and weight regain expectations, postoperative complications, and diet progression.

American Association of Endocrinologists (AACE)

www.aace.com
This site provides information on endocrine- and metabolism-related disorders (including diabetes), as well as a "find an endocrinologist" tool.

American Society for Metabolic and Bariatric Surgery (ASMBS)

http://asmbs.org
Site of an association dedicated to advancing the science of metabolic and bariatric surgeries by increasing public awareness and providing and reviewing current research.

ASMBS Integrated Health Support Group Manual

https://asmbs.org/resources/asmbs-bariatric-surgery-support-group-facilitator-manual
The *ASMBS Bariatric Surgery Support Group Facilitator Manual* is intended to help bariatric support group leaders create and provide a productive, safe, and caring environment that will allow patients and their support networks to freely express their concerns and give them an opportunity to learn from others.

Centers for Disease Control and Prevention (CDC)

www.cdc.gov
This resource provides information on obesity, heart disease, and many other conditions, as well as information on healthy eating, physical activity, and other topics.

International Federation for the Surgery of Obesity and Metabolic Disorders (IFSO)

www.ifso.com
Resources on this site include basic surgery information, videos, and current research.

Mayo Clinic

www.mayoclinic.com
This site provides information on health conditions, such as obesity, and various treatment options. It also provides links to resources for bariatric surgery.

Metabolic and Bariatric Surgery Accreditation and Quality Improvement Program (MBSAQIP)

www.facs.org/quality-programs/mbsaqip
MBSAQIP is a joint program of the American College of Surgeons (ACS) and ASMBS that provides accreditation standards for bariatric surgery centers across the nation. The site includes a standards document, "Optimal Resources for Metabolic and Bariatric Surgery 2019 Standards," which describes the pathways and standards for accreditation of metabolic and bariatric surgery centers.

National Heart, Lung, and Blood Institute (NHLBI)

www.nhlbi.nih.gov
This site features links to healthy eating resources. It includes a BMI calculator (http://nhlbisupport.com/bmi/bmicalc.htm) and apps to download for smartphones and handheld devices.

National Institute of Diabetes and Digestive and Kidney Diseases (NIDDKD)

www2.niddk.nih.gov
This resource provides information about nutrition, healthy eating, physical activity, weight control, and bariatric surgery. Many resources are available in Spanish. For information on bariatric surgery for severe obesity, go to: http://win.niddk.nih.gov/publications/PDFs/gasurg12.04bw.pdf. The NIDDK also provides information regarding the Bariatric Surgery Clinical Research Consortium, the Longitudinal Assessment of Bariatric Surgery: http://win.niddk.nih.gov/publications/PDFs/LABS_FactSheet.pdf.

Natural Medicines Database

https://naturalmedicines.therapeuticresearch.com
Natural Medicines Database uses an evidence-based approach and systematically reviews the literature to provide guidance on the safety and efficacy of food, herbs, supplements, health and wellness principles, and more.

Obesity Action Coalition (OAC)

www.obesityaction.org
The goal of this nonprofit organization is to represent and advocate for those affected by obesity. This group pushes for both legislative and educational changes and provides information on the pros and cons of bariatric surgery procedures.

Obesity Medicine Association (OMA)

https://obesitymedicine.org
OMA provides obesity medicine resources to members including obesity and algorithm and pediatric obesity algorithms and has a "find an obesity medicine clinician" search.

Office of Dietary Supplements (ODS)

http://ods.od.nih.gov
Fact sheets provide a current overview on individual vitamins, minerals, and other dietary supplements, as well as Dietary Reference Intakes and Food and Drug Administration supplement warnings and safety regulations.

The Obesity Society (TOS)

www.obesity.org
This website provides current research as well as government advocacy efforts of TOS.

UCONN Rudd Center for Food Policy and Obesity

www.uconnruddcenter.org/weight-bias-stigma
The Rudd Center aims to address weight bias and discrimination through research, education, and advocacy. Free resources are provided for clinicians and researchers to investigate and reduce weight bias, as well a free image gallery for the appropriate portrayal of individuals with obesity.

UpToDate

www.uptodate.com
This website has information about medical procedures, medications, and foods, including potential complications and drug interactions.

US Department of Agriculture My Plate

www.myplate.gov
This USDA Center for Nutrition Policy and Promotion's objectives are to advance and promote the dietary guidelines for Americans and conduct applied research in nutrition. The website provides MyPlate resources and nutrient content databases.

Weight Management Dietetic Practice Group (WM DPG)

www.wmdpg.org
WM DPG supports the highest level of professional practice in the prevention and treatment of overweight and obesity. The DPG connects the public, scientific organizations, and industry to dietetics professionals with an expertise in weight management.

APPENDIX B

Postoperative Diet Stages

Eating after metabolic and bariatric surgery is a staged approach that aims to promote healing and weight loss while minimizing the risk of gastrointestinal complications (GI). There are no standardized diet stages, but there is agreement among most institutions that a textured diet progression, from liquids to soft solids to regular textures, is best tolerated. The same diet progression can be used for sleeve gastrectomy, Roux-en-Y gastric bypass, single-anastomosis duodenal-ileostomy with sleeve, one-anastomosis gastric bypass, and biliopancreatic diversion duodenal switch. The diet progression for the adjustable gastric band (AGB) will vary slightly; differences will be noted in the sections mentioned later.

Clear Liquids

- Clear liquids can be consumed safely within hours of surgery.
- Choose clear liquids that are low in calories and sugar and are not carbonated. Caffeine may be limited or avoided in the early postoperative weeks as it is a gastric irritant.
- Clear liquid protein supplements can be incorporated to support protein needs. Without the use of clear liquid protein supplements, the clear liquid stage should not last longer than 48 hours due to nutritional inadequacy.

- Metabolic and bariatric surgeons may set a clear liquid intake goal (eg, 6 to 8 oz/h) as part of the discharge criteria. This helps ensure continued hydration after discharge.
- Encouraging patients to sip clear liquids out of 1 oz medicine cup can be helpful in the early postoperative phase. Medicine cups can help teach pacing, tracking, and goal setting for advancement and fluid intake. While straws have historically been forbidden from patient use in the early postoperative phase, there is no research that would make it a mandate to have patients avoid the use of straws after surgery. However, some patients have reported discomfort with the use of straws in the early postoperative phase, therefore, it is advised to caution patients about the use of straws and only recommend they use them if there is no GI discomfort. On the other hand, many patients report that drinking out of straws in the early postoperative phase helps them consume more fluid, therefore, preventing dehydration. It is important to work with the patient to decide what works best for them.
- Patients having AGB surgery may not require a clear liquids stage.

Full Liquids

- This stage typically begins by postoperative day 2 and lasts for 10 to 14 days. Patients having AGB surgery may only require 7 days on a full liquid diet.
- Patients should continue consuming low-calorie, noncarbonated clear liquids for hydration with a goal of at least 48 to 64 oz total fluids per day.
- Recommended full liquids are high in protein and low in added sugar. In addition to protein supplements, full liquids may include dairy or nondairy milks and smooth soups with no pieces of food. Unflavored protein powders can be added to soups to increase protein content.
- Patients may begin supplementation of vitamins and minerals in the full liquid stage. In some programs, vitamin/mineral supplementation is delayed until a soft food stage to prevent nausea from consumption of supplements on an empty stomach.

Semisolid Textures

- This stage incorporates foods with a semisolid texture, such as yogurt, cottage cheese, and ricotta cheese. It typically lasts 7 to 10 days. In some programs, these foods may be included in the full liquid diet stage.
- Some programs may refer to this stage as "pureed" or "smooth." However, if the food is soft enough for the patient to chew it well, a pureed diet may be unnecessary.
- Hydration with 48 to 64 oz clear liquid daily continues to be a priority.
- Patients will feel greater satiety with semisolid foods than with full liquids. They will likely need to eat five to six times daily, including protein supplements, to meet protein needs.
- Encourage patients to not drink with meals and to wait approximately 30 minutes after each meal before drinking fluids.
- If not yet started, patients can begin vitamin/mineral supplementation.

Soft Textures

- A soft food stage typically begins 2 to 3 weeks after surgery.
- Food textures should be soft enough to mash with a fork and for patients to thoroughly chew. Foods with skins, peels, fibrous components, and dense textures are not included in the soft foods stage.
- Hydration with 48 to 64 oz clear liquid daily continues to be a priority.
- Protein foods should be consumed first at each eating time. Patients will likely need a protein supplement as one of their eating times to meet protein needs.

Regular Textures

- Patients typically begin transitioning to regular textures 4 to 6 weeks after surgery.
- Food tolerance will vary among patients and can be impacted by texture of food as well as eating behaviors. It improves with time and tends to reach a peak at 6 months postoperatively.
- When patients begin introducing regular textures, it is common to struggle with a subset of foods that have challenging textures, such as raw fruits and vegetables, dense meats, breads, rice, and pasta.
- The diet can be communicated to patients as a nutrition "prescription" that meets nutrition needs during the rapid weight loss and healing phase. This prescription includes the following:
    - adequate hydration
    - 2 to 3 oz of protein foods three to five times a day with fruits or vegetables
    - vitamin and mineral supplementation

Band Fills/Adjustments

- The band will not be filled with saline upon initial placement. Typically, the first fill will occur 4 to 8 weeks following surgery.
- Following a fill, patients can resume full liquids for 1 to 2 days. If tolerating full liquids, patients can advance to soft foods for 4 to 5 days before resuming regular textures.
- When the diet is advanced to soft foods, it is essential that patients chew foods thoroughly since the band fill may increase the risk of improperly chewed food getting stuck above the stoma of the band.

APPENDIX C

Postoperative Metabolic Surgery Vitamin and Mineral Supplementation

Introduction

At this time, there are specific dosing recommendations for 11 different micronutrients in the prevention of micronutrient deficiencies following metabolic and bariatric surgery (MBS). The published guidelines identify varied dosing strategies for the following procedures: adjustable gastric band (AGB), sleeve gastrectomy (SG), Roux-en-Y gastric bypass (RYGB), and biliopancreatic diversion with duodenal switch (BPD/DS). Research will continue to track the long-term care of the postsurgical patient in order to further provide evidence to base future recommendations on to maximize the patients' nutritional status.

As new surgical procedures are developed and innovative medical devices are created, the practitioner should be aware of micronutrient deficiencies that commonly affect a person with obesity in order to individualize their supplement recommendations. As the science evolves, it is imperative to stay up to date with micronutrient recommendation and use clinical judgment when prevention recommendation data are not available for new surgical procedures.

Tolerable upper limits (ULs) of micronutrients have not been established for the post-MBS patient. It is important to note that some preventive micronutrient dose guidelines are higher than the general populations UL. Micronutrient toxicity in this population is not represented in the literature, although the concern is valid and should not be dismissed. The more likely nutrition consequence after surgery is a micronutrient deficiency, not toxicity. In each section mentioned later, concerns about deficiency and toxicity will be addressed.

Micronutrient Forms and Intake Methods

After surgery, there is increased risk for micronutrient deficiencies due to various factors, including the following[1]:

- Micronutrient absorption is impaired following RYGB and BPD/DS. There is a decreased interaction with intestinal absorptive surface area leading to reduced time for nutrient and enzyme interaction causing a decreased ability for nutrients to absorb.
- Reduced gastric acid production following SG can affect liberation and dissolution of vitamins and essential trace elements, especially iron and vitamin B12. Although intestinal surface area remains intact, research shows that similar long-term micronutrient deficiency rates exist when comparing SG to RYGB.
- Overall food intake and variety is reduced due to smaller stomach capacity.
- Potential food aversions or intolerances or a high intake of low-nutrient quality food choices and a low intake of high-nutrient quality foods may cause micronutrient deficiencies. See Box C.1 for general nutrient recommendations and Box C.3-C.13 for individual nutrient recommendations.

Specific Micronutrient Forms Suggested in Published Guidelines[2]

BOX C.1 Vitamin/Mineral Recommendations

Nutrient	***Recommendations***
Iron	Ferrous iron salt
	Supplemental forms with potential fewer gastrointestinal effects: heme iron polypeptide, carbonyl iron, iron amino acid chelate, or polysaccharide–iron complex
Calcium	Calcium given in divided doses
	Calcium carbonate taken with meals
	Calcium citrate taken with or without meals
Copper	Copper gluconate or sulfate is recommended source of copper for supplementation.
Folate	Folic acid or folate
Fat-soluble vitamins (A, D, E, K)	Water-miscible forms of fat-soluble vitamins improve absorption
Vitamin D	Vitamin D3 (cholecalciferol) recommended as a source for prevention of deficiency
	Vitamin D2 may be used, but additional 70% to 90% supplementation may be required for less potent form

Micronutrient Supplementation Delivery Method

In general, there is limited evidence to support the recommendation of specific delivery forms (eg, capsules, tablets, chews, and powders). While traditionally experts recommended that postsurgical patients take crushed, chewable, or liquid supplements in the immediate postoperative period (eg, first 3 to 6 months), there is lack of data to support this. Clinicians should counsel patients on the importance of taking the recommended micronutrient dose in the form that feels most comfortable to the patient.

BOX C.2 Counseling Considerations[2-6]

Prevention of micronutrient deficiencies is often easier than treatment of micronutrient deficiencies.[2]

Data continues to suggest that if patients adhere to micronutrient supplementation at recommended levels, their risk of micronutrient deficiencies is greatly decreased,[3] and that prevention of micronutrient deficiencies leads to cost savings to the patient and health care system.[4]

Data suggest that the risk of micronutrient deficiencies progresses as the length of time from surgery progresses.[2]

Data suggest that follow-up with providers and monitoring of nutritional status decrease as the length of time from surgery progresses.[5]

Education time should be spent ensuring patient understanding of the need to take micronutrient supplementation lifelong after surgery and to follow up with health care providers to ensure their nutritional status is adequate.

Work with each patient to ensure their understanding of the need to take supplements, ways to improve adherence to recommendations, and individual tolerance considerations.

The most cited reasons patients report for not taking supplements as recommended are feeling they don't need to take, forgetting to take, adverse effects, and cost.[6]

Specific Micronutrient Recommendations

Iron

Iron is a critical mineral needed for hemoglobin and myoglobin structure, as a cofactor in many proteins and redox enzymes, and is involved in many biologic processes, including lipid metabolism.[7] Absorption occurs in the duodenum and proximal jejunum and depends on individual host factors, with iron stores having the greatest influence.[8] Additional factors that may affect absorption include the source of iron and other dietary or supplemental inhibitors (eg, minerals such as calcium, tannins, polyphenols, phytates, and acid-reducing medications) or enhancers (eg, vitamin C and presence of meat consumption).

Deficiency can lead to significant morbidity including fatigue, hair loss, brittle nails, angular cheilosis, and anemia. It can also impact the underlying pulmonary or cardiovascular disease.[1] Diminished stomach acid production occurs with SG, RYGB, and BPD/DS, and bypassing of the duodenum in RYGB or BPD/DS leads to significant deficiency rates in postoperative patients, with the exception of the AGB, which has low reported rates of iron deficiency.[1,7]

- Iron deficiency can often be avoided with adherence to appropriate nutrition and a high-quality multivitamin supplement that contains the recommended prevention dose.[7] However, the risk may not be entirely eliminated, and patients should be screened lifelong after all procedures.
- Individual tolerance of iron supplements varies. Patients who require large doses of iron may need to try different forms to assess tolerance level.
- Instruct patient to take supplements containing iron with meals (see the following for nutrient inhibitors) to alleviate potential gastrointestinal (GI) distress.

- Take separately[2,7] from high-calcium food sources or supplements, acid-reducing medications, and foods high in phytates or polyphenols to maximize absorption potential.
- If patient needs more than the prevention doses listed later, it is recommended to take in divided doses throughout the day (ie, 65 mg elemental iron BID-TID).

BOX C.3 Iron Recommendations[1,2,9,10]

Adjustable gastric banding	
Preoperative deficiency rates	8% to 45%
Postoperative deficiency rates (more than 12 months)	0% to 32%
Daily recommended prevention dose	At least 18 mg
Sleeve gastrectomy	
Preoperative deficiency rates	8% to 45%
Postoperative deficiency rates (more than 12 months)	15% to 45%
Daily recommended prevention dose	At least 45 to 60 mg
Roux-en-Y gastric bypass	
Preoperative deficiency rates	8% to 45%
Postoperative deficiency rates (more than 12 months)	25% to 50%
Daily recommended prevention dose	At least 45 to 60 mg
Biliopancreatic diversion with duodenal switch	
Preoperative deficiency rates	8% to 45%
Postoperative deficiency rates (more than 12 months)	25%
Daily recommended prevention dose	At least 45 to 60 mg

Vitamin B12 and Folate (B9)

Vitamin B12, a water-soluble vitamin, is needed for proper function of the brain and nervous system, red blood cell maturation, neural function, and DNA formation.[11] Folate (food-derived) and folic acid (synthetic) are forms of vitamin B9 needed for cellular division, nucleic acid synthesis, amino acid metabolism, and neurotransmitter production.[12]

There is a synergistic effect between folate and vitamin B12, as both play a role in DNA synthesis, cellular metabolism, prevention of cardiovascular disease and cognitive functioning, and in the conversion of homocysteine to methionine—an amino acid that plays an essential role in metabolism and health.[11] Over supplementation of folate can mask a potential vitamin B12 deficiency, and a vitamin B12 deficiency may cause folate deficiency. The practitioner should educate the patient on proper dosing for each of these micronutrients due to their connected relationship in the body.

A deficiency in vitamin B12 or folate can lead to megaloblastic macrocytic anemia. Symptoms of vitamin B12 deficiency include numbness or tingling in fingers and toes, glossitis, fatigue, depression, dementia, gait ataxia, and elevated homocysteine levels. Symptoms of folate deficiency include changes in skin and nail pigmentation, oral mucosal ulcerations, and elevated homocysteine levels.

- Active absorption of vitamin B12 is dependent on hydrochloric acid (to release food-bound vitamin B12) and intrinsic factor (a glycoprotein that binds to vitamin B12 to enable absorption in the small intestine), which are both secreted by parietal cells in the stomach.
- When vitamin B12 is ingested after surgical procedures that either decrease the body's ability to mix with these substrates (RYGB, SG, BPD/DS) or remove a majority of the cells that produce them (SG)—approximately 1% of vitamin B12 can be absorbed via passive diffusion.
- In purely restrictive procedures, vitamin B12 deficiency is not as common; however, note that aging is an independent risk factor for vitamin B12 deficiency. If protein intolerance is evident or the patient takes medications that can affect vitamin B12 status (eg, protein pump inhibitors), they may still have an elevated risk of deficiency.

- Vitamin B12 is stored in the liver. The average adult has storage available for multiple years. However, the typical absorption pathway cannot occur after most MBS procedures, and irreversible nerve damage can occur with an undiagnosed vitamin B12 deficiency. Therefore, long-term deficiency risk should not be dismissed.[11]
- Serum vitamin B12 is sensitive to recent intake. If patient has an elevated level, screen for timing of supplementation prior to laboratory draw, review methylmalonic acid (MMA) or homocysteine if available, and counsel patient on appropriate daily intake of vitamin B12 (including all supplements and fortified foods or beverages).
- Practitioner discretion should guide counseling recommendations. Potential interventions could include to repeat laboratory draw with instruction of fasting from supplements prior to laboratory draw, stop additional vitamin B12 (if patient was taking dose above or below recommendations), and repeat laboratory in 1 month. If clinician advises to stop B12 supplementation, it is imperative that they emphasize the importance of follow-up laboratory draws to assess trends lifelong, ensure the patient understands that they will likely need to restart supplementation.
- Folate is essential for the prevention of fetal neural tube defects. For patients who are of childbearing age, careful attention should be placed on proper folate/folic acid consumption.
- Folate is stored in the liver but only in small amounts. Absorption of folate and folic acid after most MBS procedures does not seem to be hindered as the active site for absorption is the jejunum, and it can be absorbed passively along the small intestine.
- Risk of folate deficiency is higher in a patient nonadherent to micronutrient supplementation, has a low intake of folate-rich foods, high intake of alcohol, or takes medications that interfere with folate absorption.
- Folic acid supplementation above 1 mg (1,700 mcg dietary folate equivalent [DFE]) per day is not recommended due to the potential to mask a vitamin B12 deficiency.

BOX C.4 Vitamin B12 Recommendations[1,2,9,10]

Adjustable gastric banding	
Preoperative deficiency rates	2% to 30%
Postoperative deficiency rates (more than12 months)	10%
Daily recommended prevention dose	350 to 500 mcg oral, tablet, sublingual, liquid, or nasal, as directed Or 1,000 mcg/mo intramuscular injection or subqutaneous
Sleeve gastrectomy	
Preoperative deficiency rates	2% to 30%
Postoperative deficiency rates (more than12 months)	10% to 20%
Daily recommended prevention dose	350 to 500 mcg oral, tablet, sublingual, liquid, or nasal, as directed or 1,000 mcg/mo, IM or SQ
Roux-en-Y gastric bypass	
Preoperative deficiency rates	2% to 30%
Postoperative deficiency rates (more than12 months)	30% to 50%
Daily recommended prevention dose	350 to 500 mcg oral, tablet, sublingual, liquid, or nasal, as directed or 1,000 mcg/mo, IM or SQ

BOX C.4 Vitamin B12 Recommendations[1,2,9,10] (cont.)

Biliopancreatic diversion with duodenal switch

Preoperative deficiency rates	2% to 30%
Postoperative deficiency rates (more than12 months)	22%
Daily recommended prevention dose	350 to 500 mcg oral, tablet, sublingual, liquid, or nasal, as directed or 1,000 mcg/mo,F IM or SQ

BOX C.5 Folate Recommendations[a,1,2,9,10]

Adjustable gastric banding

Preoperative deficiency rates	Up to 54%
Postoperative deficiency rates (more than12 months)	10%
Daily recommended prevention dose	400 to 800 mcg 800 to 1,000 mcg females of childbearing age 2020 supplement label: • 1,335 mcg dietary folate equivalent (DFE) = 800 mcg folic acid • 1 mcg DFE = 1 mcg folate • 1 mcg DFE = 0.6 mcg folic acid

Sleeve gastrectomy

Preoperative deficiency rates	Up to 54%
Postoperative deficiency rates (more than12 months)	10% to 20%

Continued on next page

BOX C.5 Folate Recommendations[1,2,9,10] (cont.)

Daily recommended prevention dose	400 to 800 mcg 800 to 1,000 mcg females of childbearing age 2020 supplement label: • 1,335 mcg (DFE = 800 mcg folic acid • 1 mcg DFE = 1 mcg folate • 1 mcg DFE = 0.6 mcg folic acid
Roux-en-Y gastric bypass	
Preoperative deficiency rates	Up to 54%
Postoperative deficiency rates (more than12 months)	15%
Daily recommended prevention dose	400 to 800 mcg 800 to 1,000 mcg females of childbearing age 2020 supplement label: • 1,335 mcg DFE = 800 mcg folic acid • 1 mcg DFE = 1 mcg folate • 1 mcg DFE = 0.6 mcg folic acid
Biliopancreatic diversion with duodenal switch	
Preoperative deficiency rates	Up to 54%
Postoperative deficiency rates (after 12 months)	15%
Daily recommended prevention dose	400 to 800 mcg 800 to 1,000 mcg females of childbearing age 2020 supplement label: • 1,335 mcg DFE = 800 mcg folic acid • 1 mcg DFE = 1 mcg folate • 1 mcg DFE = 0.6 mcg folic acid

[a] Specific recommendations for transgender and gender-diverse people were not provided.

Zinc and Copper

Zinc is a trace element that is needed for DNA synthesis, wound healing, taste acuity, and protein synthesis—more than 300 proteins and more than 1,000 transcription factors utilize zinc.[13] Absorption occurs in the duodenum and proximal jejunum, where it competes with absorption with copper. There are no large body stores of zinc, so careful attention should be paid to intake.[13] Copper is a trace metal that is essential for iron absorption and neurotransmitter synthesis and is absorbed in the stomach and duodenum.

- Zinc deficiency can lead to hair loss, glossitis, delayed wound healing, decreased taste sensations, impaired folate absorption, and skin lesions.[13]
- Copper deficiency can lead to anemia, neutropenia, optic neuropathy, fatigue, and iron deficiency.[1]
- Zinc and copper deficiencies can typically be avoided with adherence to appropriate nutrition and a high-quality multivitamin supplement.[7]
- Due to intestinal competition for absorption and since high intakes of zinc induce biliary excretion of copper, a ratio of 8 to 15 mg of elemental zinc to 1 mg copper is recommended.[2,9]

BOX C.6 Zinc Recommendations[a,1,2,9,10]

Adjustable gastric banding

Preoperative deficiency rates	24% to 74%
Postoperative deficiency rates (after 12 months)	Up to 34%
Daily recommended prevention dose	8 to 11 mg based on Recommended Dietary Allowance (RDA) • Male: 11 mg/d • Female: 8 mg/d

Continued on next page

BOX C.6 Zinc Recommendations[1,2,9,10] (cont.)

Sleeve gastrectomy

Preoperative deficiency rates	24% to 74%
Postoperative deficiency rates (after 12 months)	Up to 19%
Daily recommended prevention dose	8 to 11 mg based on RDA • Male: 11 mg/d • Female: 8 mg/d

Roux-en-Y gastric bypass

Preoperative deficiency rates	24% to 74%
Postoperative deficiency rates (after 12 months)	Up to 40%
Daily recommended prevention dose	8 to 22 mg based on RDA • Male: 11 to 22 mg/d • Female: 8 to 16 mg/d

Biliopancreatic diversion with duodenal switch

Preoperative deficiency rates	24% to 74%
Postoperative deficiency rates (after 12 months)	Up to 70%
Daily recommended prevention dose	16 to 22 mg based on RDA • Male: 22 mg/d • Female: 16 mg/d

[a] Specific recommendations for transgender and gender-diverse people were not provided.

BOX C.7 Copper Recommendations[a,1,2,9,10]

Adjustable gastric banding

Preoperative deficiency rates	Limited data, with the exception of pre–biliopancreatic diversion (BPD) females: up to 70%
Postoperative deficiency rates (after 12 months)	Not reported
Daily recommended prevention dose	1 mg

Sleeve gastrectomy

Preoperative deficiency rates	Limited data, with the exception of pre-BPD females: up to 70%
Postoperative deficiency rates (after 12 months)	10%
Daily recommended prevention dose	1 mg

Roux-en-Y gastric bypass

Preoperative deficiency rates	Limited data, with the exception of pre-BPD females: up to 70%
Postoperative deficiency rates (after 12 months)	10%
Daily recommended prevention dose	2 mg

Biliopancreatic diversion with duodenal switch

Preoperative deficiency rates	Limited data, with the exception of pre-BPD females: up to 70%
Postoperative deficiency rates (after 12 months)	70%
Daily recommended prevention dose	2 mg

[a] Specific recommendations for transgender and gender-diverse people were not provided.

Vitamin D and Calcium

Vitamin D is an essential fat-soluble micronutrient that is needed for calcium metabolism, bone health, neuromuscular functioning, and immune health. In the absence of adequate vitamin D status, calcium (and phosphorus) absorption is greatly decreased.[14] Calcium is an important mineral that is involved in bone and tooth formation, blood coagulation, muscle contraction, nerve conduction, and hormonal secretion.

- Vitamin D deficiency may lead to decreased bone mineralization, osteopenia, and secondary hyperparathyroidism.
- Vitamin D deficiency or insufficiency is common in patients with overweight and obesity regardless of surgical status.
- Calcium deficiency can be a challenge to identify as serum calcium levels are tightly regulated and will remain within normal limits (in the absence of kidney disease).
- Calcium deficiency can lead to decreased bone mineralization, osteopenia, and secondary hyperparathyroidism.

BOX C.8 Vitamin D Recommendations[1,2,9,10]

Adjustable gastric banding	
Preoperative deficiency rates	Up to 100%
Postoperative deficiency rates (more than12 months)	30%
Daily recommended prevention dose	At least 3,000 IU Maintain 25-hydroxyvitamin D levels higher than 30 ng/mL 2020 supplement label: • 75 mcg = 3,000 IU • 0.025 mcg = 1 IU
Sleeve gastrectomy	
Preoperative deficiency rates	Up to 100%
Postoperative deficiency rates (more than12 months)	30% to 70%

BOX C.8 Vitamin D Recommendations[1,2,9,10] (cont.)

Daily recommended prevention dose	At least 3,000 IU Maintain 25-hydroxyvitamin D levels higher than30 ng/mL 2020 supplement label: • 75 mcg = 3,000 IU • 0.025 mcg = 1 IU

Roux-en-Y gastric bypass

Preoperative deficiency rates	Up to 100%
Postoperative deficiency rates (more than12 months)	30% to 50%
Daily recommended prevention dose	At least 3,000 IU Maintain 25-hydroxyvitamin D levels more than 30 ng/mL 2020 supplement label: • 75 mcg = 3,000 IU • 0.025 mcg = 1 IU

Biliopancreatic diversion with duodenal switch

Preoperative deficiency rates	Up to 100%
Postoperative deficiency rates (more than12 months)	40% to 100%
Daily recommended prevention dose	At least 3,000 IU Maintain 25-hydroxyvitamin D levels higher than30 ng/mL 2020 supplement label: • 75 mcg = 3,000 IU • 0.025 mcg = 1 IU

BOX C.9 Calcium Recommendations[1,2,9,10]

Adjustable gastric banding

Preoperative deficiency rates	Difficult to identify
Postoperative deficiency rates (more than12 months)	Difficult to identify
Daily recommended prevention dose	1,200 to 1,500 mg

Sleeve gastrectomy

Preoperative deficiency rates	Difficult to identify
Postoperative deficiency rates (more than12 months)	Difficult to identify
Daily recommended prevention dose	1,200 to 1,500 mg

Roux-en-Y gastric bypass

Preoperative deficiency rates	Difficult to identify
Postoperative deficiency rates (more than12 months)	Difficult to identify
Daily recommended prevention dose	1,200 to 1,500 mg

Biliopancreatic diversion with duodenal switch

Preoperative deficiency rates	Difficult to identify
Postoperative deficiency rates (more than12 months)	Difficult to identify
Daily recommended prevention dose	1,800 to 2,400 mg

Vitamin A

Vitamin A is an essential fat-soluble micronutrient made of a group of carotenoids and retinoids that act as antioxidants and function as cofactors in vision, immune function, and connective tissue maintenance. Lipid digestion is delayed after RYGB and BPD/DS, as nutrients do not pass through the duodenum, which limits the interaction with bile and pancreatic lipase, placing these patients at greater risk for fat-soluble vitamin deficiencies. As with all fat-soluble nutrients, vitamin A must be incorporated into a micelle for absorption. Any procedure that decreases micelle production or delays food or supplemental intake with micelles in the small intestine has greater risk of vitamin A deficiency.

- Vitamin A is involved in hemoglobin production and can affect anemia.
- Vitamin A deficiency can lead to night blindness, Bitot spots, poor wound healing, hyperkeratinization of the skin, and loss of taste.
- Ingestion of preformed vitamin A (eg, retinol) above levels of 10,000 IU per day is not recommended as the liver stores vitamin A with limited excretion. Large intakes of provitamin A (eg, carotenoids) are not associated with toxicity risk.[15]
- In general, it is recommended that supplements containing vitamin A are a blend of retinol sources and carotenoid sources.

BOX C.10 Vitamin A Recommendations[1,2,9,10]

Adjustable gastric banding

Preoperative deficiency rates	14%
Postoperative deficiency rates (more than12 months)	10%
Daily recommended prevention dose	5,000 IU

Continued on next page

BOX C.10 Vitamin A Recommendations[1,2,9,10] (cont.)

Sleeve gastrectomy

Preoperative deficiency rates	14%
Postoperative deficiency rates (more than12 months)	10% to 20%
Daily recommended prevention dose	5,000 to 10,000 IU 2020 supplement label listed in Retinol Activity Equivalent (RAE): • 1 mcg RAE = 1 mcg retinol • 1 mcg RAE = 2 mcg supplemental beta carotene • 1 IU = 0.3 mcg retinol • 1 IU = 0.6 mcg β carotene

Roux-en-Y gastric bypass

Preoperative deficiency rates	14%
Postoperative deficiency rates (more than12 months)	10% to 50%
Daily recommended prevention dose	5,000 to 10,000 IU 2020 supplement label listed in RAE: • 1 mcg RAE = 1 mcg retinol • 1 mcg RAE = 2 mcg supplemental β carotene • 1 IU = 0.3 mcg retinol • 1 IU = 0.6 mcg β carotene

Biliopancreatic diversion with duodenal switch

Preoperative deficiency rates	14%
Postoperative deficiency rates (more than12 months)	60% to 70%
Daily recommended prevention dose	10,000 IU

Vitamins E and K

Vitamin E is an essential fat-soluble micronutrient that acts as an antioxidant and is needed for enzyme production, gene expressions, and neurological functions.[7] Fat-soluble deficiencies, including vitamin E, are more likely to occur following highly malabsorptive procedures like the BPD/DS due to the nature of fat-soluble vitamin absorption. Vitamin K is essential for blood clot formation and bone metabolism and is rare in the general population and not reported after MBS procedures. However, the risk may still be present after any alteration in the GI tract.

- Vitamin E deficiency may cause neuropathy and ataxia, gait disturbances, or muscle weakness.
- Vitamin K deficiency may cause bruising and uncontrolled bleeding, bleeding gums, or delayed blood clotting.

BOX C.11 Vitamin E Recommendations[1,2,9,10]

Adjustable gastric banding

Preoperative deficiency rates	Uncommon
Postoperative deficiency rates (more than12 months)	0%
Daily recommended prevention dose	15 mg 2020 supplement label listed in mg of α-tocopherol: • 1 IU = 0.67 mg for *d*-α-tocopherol (natural) • 1 IU = 0.9 mg for *dl*-α-tocopherol (synthetic) • 1 mg vitamin E label claim = 1 mg of natural α-tocopherol • 1 mg vitamin E label claim = 2 mg of synthetic α-tocopherol

Continued on next page

BOX C.11 Vitamin E Recommendations[1,2,9,10] (cont.)

Sleeve gastrectomy

Preoperative deficiency rates	Uncommon
Postoperative deficiency rates (more than12 months)	0% to 5%
Daily recommended prevention dose	15 mg 2020 supplement label listed in mg of α-tocopherol: • 1 IU = 0.67 mg for *d*-α-tocopherol (natural) • 1 IU = 0.9 mg for *dl*-α-tocopherol (synthetic) • 1 mg vitamin E label claim = 1 mg of natural α-tocopherol • 1 mg vitamin E label claim = 2 mg of synthetic α-tocopherol

Roux-en-Y gastric bypass

Preoperative deficiency rates	Uncommon
Postoperative deficiency rates (more than12 months)	10%
Daily recommended prevention dose	15 mg 2020 supplement label listed in mg of α-tocopherol: • 1 IU = 0.67 mg for *d*-α-tocopherol (natural) • 1 IU = 0.9 mg for *dl*-α-tocopherol (synthetic) • 1 mg vitamin E label claim = 1 mg of natural α-tocopherol • 1 mg vitamin E label claim = 2 mg of synthetic α-tocopherol

BOX C.11 Vitamin E Recommendations[1,2,9,10] (cont.)

Biliopancreatic diversion with duodenal switch

Preoperative deficiency rates	Uncommon
Postoperative deficiency rates (more than12 months)	10%
Daily recommended prevention dose	15 mg 2020 supplement label listed in mg of α-tocopherol: • 1 IU = 0.67 mg for *d*-α-tocopherol (natural) • 1 IU = 0.9 mg for *dl*-α-tocopherol (synthetic) • 1 mg vitamin E label claim = 1 mg of natural α-tocopherol • 1 mg vitamin E label claim = 2 mg of synthetic α-tocopherol

BOX C.12 Vitamin K Recommendations[1,2,9,10]

Adjustable gastric banding

Preoperative deficiency rates	Not reported
Postoperative deficiency rates (more than 12 months)	0
Daily recommended prevention dose	90 to 120 mcg

Sleeve gastrectomy

Preoperative deficiency rates	Not reported
Postoperative deficiency rates (more than12 months)	0
Daily recommended prevention dose	90 to 120 mcg

Continued on next page

BOX C.12 Vitamin K Recommendations[1,2,9,10] (cont.)

Roux-en-Y gastric bypass	
Preoperative deficiency rates	Not reported
Postoperative deficiency rates (more than12 months)	0%
Daily recommended prevention dose	90 to 120 mcg
Biliopancreatic diversion with duodenal switch	
Preoperative deficiency rates	Not reported
Postoperative deficiency rates (more than12 months)	60% to 70%
Daily recommended prevention dose	300 mcg

Vitamin B1 (Thiamin)

Thiamin is an essential water-soluble micronutrient that is an enzymatic cofactor involved in multiple cellular processes including glycolysis, the citric acid cycle, amino acid synthesis, the pentose phosphate shunt pathway, and neurotransmitter synthesis. Deficiency of thiamin impairs oxidative metabolism, which can lead to inflammation, oxidative stress, and neurodegeneration.[16] Thiamin absorption is dependent on hydrolysis and enzymatic phosphatase that is found in the proximal intestine, which puts SG, RYGB, and BPD/DS patients at the greatest risk for deficiency.[2]

- Thiamin deficiency can lead to nausea and vomiting, neuropathy, gait ataxia, and confusion.
- Thiamin deficiency can cause wet or dry beriberi and Wernicke encephalopathy.[17]
- Risk of thiamin deficiency may be increased with prolonged vomiting, rapid weight loss, excessive carbohydrate intake, and alcoholism.

BOX C.13 Thiamin Recommendations[1,2,9,10]

Adjustable gastric banding

Preoperative deficiency rates	As high as 29%
Postoperative deficiency rates (more than12 months)	0%
Daily recommended prevention dose	At least 12 mg
	High-risk patients: 50 to 100 mg

Sleeve gastrectomy

Preoperative deficiency rates	As high as 29%
Postoperative deficiency rates (more than12 months)	0%
Daily recommended prevention dose	At least 12 mg
	High-risk patients: 50 to 100 mg

Roux-en-Y gastric bypass

Preoperative deficiency rates	As high as 29%
Postoperative deficiency rates (more than12 months)	12%
Daily recommended prevention dose	At least 12 mg
	High-risk patients: 50 to 100 mg

Biliopancreatic diversion with duodenal switch

Preoperative deficiency rates	As high as 29%
Postoperative deficiency rates (more than12 months)	10% to 15%
Daily recommended prevention dose	At least 12 mg
	High-risk patients: 50 to 100 mg

Additional Micronutrient Considerations

In addition to the 11 micronutrients listed earlier, published guidelines suggest that patients who have had an bariatric surgery take a multivitamin that contains trace minerals including selenium and magnesium and that they receive 100% to 200% of the daily value of all B vitamins or an optional B50 complex daily.[2,18]

Micronutrient supplementation should always focus on the minimum preventive dose as suggested by MBS published guidelines and should be discussed with the registered dietitian nutritionist (RDN) at each visit. To achieve these high levels of micronutrient intake, patients may choose to purchase specialized bariatric micronutrient supplements to decrease their daily pill burden, which has been shown to improve adherence to recommendations.

Conclusion

Prevention of micronutrient deficiencies is of utmost importance after MBS and should be a major focus of the entire bariatric interdisciplinary team. However, the responsibility often lies primarily on the RDN. It is important to follow serum makers, physical signs and symptoms, and assess for adherence to appropriate micronutrient supplementation for all patients to ensure their nutrition status is normal after surgery.

References

1. Via MA, Mechanick JI. Nutritional and micronutrient care of bariatric surgery patients: current evidence update. *Curr Obes Rep.* 2017;6:286-296. doi:10.1007/s13679-017-0271-x
2. Parrott J, Frank L, Rabena R, et al. American Society for Metabolic and Bariatric Surgery Integrated Health Nutritional Guidelines for the Surgical Weight Loss Patient—2016 update: micronutrients. *Surg Obes Relat Dis.* 2016;12:955-959. doi:10.1016/j.soard.2016.12.018

3. Schijns W, Schuurman LT, Melse-Boonstra A, et al. Do specialized bariatric multivitamins lower deficiencies after RYGB? *Surg Obes Relat Dis.* 2018;14(7):1005-1012. doi:10.1016/j.soard.2018.03.029
4. Homan J, Schijns W, Janssen IMC, Berends FJ, Aarts EO. Adequate multivitamin supplementation after Roux-en-Y gastric bypass results in a decrease of national health care costs: a cost-effectiveness analysis. *Obes Surg.* 2019;29:1638-1643. doi:10.1007/s11695-019-03750-6
5. Fox W, Borgert A, Rasmussen C, et al. Long-term micronutrient surveillance after gastric bypass surgery in an integrated healthcare system. *Surg Obes Relat Dis.* 2019;15(3):389-395. doi:10.1016/j.soard.2018.12.029
6. Smelt HJM, Pouwels S, Smulders JF, Hazebroek EJ. Patient adherence to multivitamin supplementation after bariatric surgery: a narrative review. *J Nutr Sci.* 2020;9:e46. doi:10.1017/jns.2020.41
7. Bays HE, Jones PH, Jacobson TA, et al. Lipids and bariatric procedures part 1 of 2: scientific statement from the National Lipid Association, American Society for Metabolic and Bariatric Surgery, and Obesity Medicine Association: executive summary. *J Clin Lipidol.* 2016;10(1):15-32. doi:10.1016/j.jacl.2015.12.003
8. Chan LN, Mike LA. The science and practice of micronutrient supplementations in nutritional anemia: an evidence-based review. *J Parenter Enteral Nutr.* 2014;38(6):656-672. doi:10.1177/0148607114533726
9. Mechanick JI, Apovian C, Brethaur S, et al. Clinical practice guidelines for the perioperative nutrition, metabolic, and nonsurgical support of patients undergoing bariatric procedures—2019 update: cosponsored by American Association of Clinical Endocrinologists/American College of Endocrinology, the Obesity Society, American Society for Metabolic & Bariatric Surgery, Obesity Medicine Association, and American Society of Anesthesiologists. *Surg Obes Relat Dis.* 2020;16(2):175-247. doi:10.4158/GL-2019-0406
10. Stein J, Stier C, Raab H, Weiner R. Review article: the nutritional and pharmacological consequences of obesity surgery. *Al Pharm Ther.* 2014;40:582-609. doi:10.1111/apt.12872
11. O'Leary F, Samman S. Vitamin B12 in health and disease. *Nutrients.* 2010;2(3):299-316. doi:10.3390/nu2030299
12. Caudill MA. Folate bioavailability: implications for establishing dietary recommendations and optimizing status. *Am J Clin Nutr.* 2010;91:1455S-1460S. doi:10.3945/ajcn.2010.28674E
13. Livingstone C. Zinc: physiology, deficiency, and parenteral nutrition. *Nutr Clin Pract.* 2015;30(3):371-382. doi:10.1177/0884533615570376

Appendixes

14. Holick MF, Binkley NC, Bischoff-Ferrari HA, et al. Evaluation, treatment, and prevention of vitamin D deficiency: an Endocrine Society Clinical Practice Guideline. *J Clin Endocrinol.* 2011;96:1911-1930. doi:10.1210/jc.2011-0385

15. Grune T, Lietz G, Palou A, et al. Beta-carotene is an important vitamin A source for humans. *J Nutr.* 2010;140(12):2268S-2285S. doi:10.3945/jn.109.119024

16. Liu D, Ke Z, Luo J. Thiamine deficiency and neurodegeneration: the interplay among oxidative stress, endoplasmic reticulum stress, and autophagy. *Mol Neurobiol.* 2017;54:5440-5448. doi:10.1007/s12035-016-0079-9

17. Matrana MR, Vasireddy S, Davis WE. The skinny on a growing problem: dry beriberi after bariatric surgery. *Ann Intern Med.* 2008;149(11):842-844. doi:10.7326/0003-4819-149-11-200812020-00026

18. Aills L, Blankenship J, Buffington C, Furtado M, Parrott J. ASMBS allied health nutritional guidelines for the surgical weight loss patient. *Surg Obes Relat Dis.* 2008;4:S73-S108. doi:10.1016/j.soard.2008.03.002

APPENDIX D

Biochemical Surveillance After Metabolic and Bariatric Surgery

Over time, postoperative micronutrient deficiencies increase while monitoring of potential deficiencies decreases.[1,2]

Surveillance Schedule

The metabolic and bariatric surgery (MBS) care team, including the registered dietitian nutritionists (RDNs), should monitor nutrition-related laboratory values for all patients who have had an MBS at a minimum of annually. Prior to laboratory draw, it is reasonable to recommend abstaining from supplement intake for at least 8 hours, as some nutritional markers are influenced by recent supplemental intake; however, there are limited data to support this guidance.

Preoperative Repletion of Nutrient Deficiencies

Experts recommend that all preoperative deficiencies be repleted and confirmed with laboratory assessment before MBS surgery.[2] Table D.1 lists the nutrition-related laboratory markers to be assessed. Preoperative repletion recommendations is an area of study that has limited data. The RDN should provide individualized guidance based on the patients' laboratory values, risk factors, time to surgery, and other individual considerations (eg, gender, degree of deficiency, age).

There are clinical limitations to some patients receiving a full nutrition screen prior to surgery. While not ideal, patients can begin on postoperative prevention dose supplementation (see Appendix C) prior to surgery in an effort to attempt to correct unidentified preoperative deficiencies.[4]

Postoperative Repletion of Nutrient Deficiencies

Overview

It is important to remember that micronutrients work synergistically. When one is deficient, it will likely negatively affect another micronutrient.

TABLE D.1 Biochemical Surveillance Schedule for Patients Who Have Had Bariatric Surgery[2-7]

	Presurgery	Within 3 months postoperative	Every 3 to 6 months in the first year postoperative	Annually	Marker(s)
Lipid panel	✓	✓	✓	✓	
Kidney function	✓	✓	✓	✓	
Liver profile	✓	✓	✓	✓	
Complete blood count	✓	✓	✓	✓	
Thyroid-stimulating hormone	✓	As needed	As needed	As needed	
Hemoglobin A1c[a]	✓	As needed	As needed	As needed	
Dual energy x-ray absorptiometry, bone density				✓ (every 2 years)	

Continued on next page

TABLE D.1 Biochemical Surveillance Schedule for Patients Who Have Had Bariatric Surgery[2-7] (cont.)

	Presurgery	Within 3 months postoperative	Every 3 to 6 months in the first year postoperative	Annually	Marker(s)
Iron	✓	✓	✓	✓	Ferritin with c-reactive protein; full iron panel (iron, transferrin, % saturation, total iron-binding capacity)
Thiamin	✓	✓	✓	✓	Whole blood thiamine (thiamine pyrophosphate)
Folate	✓		✓	✓	Serum folate, red blood cell folate, homocysteine
Vitamin B12	✓	✓?	✓	✓	Serum B12, methylmalonic acid
Vitamin D	✓		✓	✓	25-hydroxyvitamin D, intact parathyroid hormone
Calcium	✓		✓	✓	Ionized calcium

Vitamin A	Optional	✓ 1 x w/in first year	Roux-en-Y gastric bypass (RYGB) Biliopancreatic diversion with duodenal switch (BPD/DS)	Serum vitamin A, retinol-binding protein, plasma retinol
Vitamins E, K	Optional		RYGB BPD/DS	Plasma α-tocopherol, des-gamma-carboxy prothrombin, prothrombin time/international normalized ratio, serum vitamin K
Zinc			✓	Plasma or serum zinc, red blood cell zinc
Copper			RYGB BPD/DS Sleeve gas-trectomy with symptoms	Serum copper, ceruloplasmin with c-reactive protein

Key: ✓ = test for all procedures unless otherwise indicated; ✓? = test is not necessary unless indicated by physical assessment findings or patients at high risk for deficiency.

[a] Evaluate hemoglobin A1c (HbA1c) in patients with suspected or diagnosed prediabetes or diabetes. Preoperative testing is optional but advisable for all patients, with goal of HbA1c of 7% to 8% or less before surgery to reduce risk of complications.

When there is a serum marker confirmation of a micronutrient deficiency, follow the repletion recommendations mentioned later until the serum marker is found to be within normal limits (WNLs), then resume prevention dose guidelines. It can also be useful to assess trends of serum markers when available, not simply one laboratory draw.

If feasible, monitor nutrient status often (eg, every 3 months) until a series of consecutive laboratory draws indicate that the deficiency is corrected and stable. Also, ensure that high risk factors that may have potentially contributed to the deficiency state (ie, protein-calorie malnutrition) have been reduced. Some patients will need higher than normal prevention levels of certain micronutrients lifelong to prevent deficiency states and will need to be followed more closely.

Performing a nutrition-focused physical examination is also recommended to assess for physical signs and symptoms of deficiencies. When assessing a patient, it can be helpful for the practitioner to think in terms of bodily systems or functions to assess for states of deficiency. For example, questions around energy levels can help assess for anemias, while questions related to cognitive function (eg, memory) can help identify neurological disorders. Another assessment strategy would be a "head-to-toe" approach, observing or asking questions related to a patient's hair, skin, eyes, mouth/tongue, nails, gait, and so on. See Appendix C for advice on supplement regimens.

BOX D.1 Nutrition-Related Laboratory Assessment and Related Interventions After Metabolic and Bariatric Surgery: Anemias[2-9]

Iron	
Risk factors for deficiency	Preexisting deficiency, malabsorptive surgery, menstruation, excessive blood loss, chronic gastronintestinal blood loss, diverticulosis, insufficient supplementation, avoidance of meat, copper deficiency
Serum marker(s)	↓Ferritin (or within normal limits [WNLs] ferritin with ↑c-reactive protein [CRP]), transferrin saturation, iron, mean corpuscular volume *Low ferritin cut off w/ CRP value:* If CRP <5 mcg/L; ferritin low = <30 mcg/L If CRP ≥5 mcg/L; ferritin low = <100 mcg/L ↑Transferrin iron-binding capacity, transferrin soluble receptor zinc protoporphyrin
Physical signs and symptoms	Fatigue, low productivity, spoon-shaped nails, vertical ridges on nails, glossitis, smooth shiny tongue
Oral repletion (per day unless indicated)	Iron depletion (stage I/II iron status) or high-risk patients: 50 to 100 mg elemental iron Iron deficiency (stage III/IV iron status): 150 to 200 mg elemental iron up to 300 mg two to three times per day Unable to tolerate oral iron or not responding: intravenous iron may be required (comes in different formulations, some require a test dose)
Vitamin B12	
Risk factors for deficiency	Malabsorptive surgery, decreased meat and dairy intake, rapid weight loss, low food intake, alcoholism, irritable bowel syndrome, use of metformin or proton pump inhibitors, insufficient supplementation

Continued on next page

BOX D.1 Nutrition-Related Laboratory Assessment and Related Interventions After Metabolic and Bariatric Surgery: Anemias[2-9] (cont.)

Serum marker(s)	↑ Serum methylmalonic acid (MMA), mean corpuscular volume, homocysteine ↓ Serum B12
Physical signs and symptoms	Numbness/tingling fingers and toes, pale skin, fatigue, depression, dementia, gait ataxia, glossitis, red beefy tongue
Oral repletion (per day unless indicated)	1,000 mcg (stage III to IV vitamin B12 status): *Note: Postoperative deficiency studies indicate oral vitamin B12 at high enough doses can efficiently correct deficiency*
	Note: Can receive 1,000 mcg/month intramuscular injection if unresponsive to oral
Folate	
Risk factors for deficiency	Low intake (vegetarianism), vitamin B6 or B12 deficiencies, insufficient supplementation or low adherence with supplementation
Serum marker(s)	↑ Homocysteine ↓ Red blood cell folate (WNL MMA) Urinary formiminoglutamic acid
Physical signs and symptoms	Fatigue, changes in skin pigmentation, risk of neural tube defects in fetus
Oral repletion (per day unless indicated)	1,000 mcg (stage III/IV folate status) *Note: If multivitamin contains 400 mcg folic acid, okay to add 800 mcg folic acid (total 1.2 mg per day) until normal range reached; long-term use of 1,000 mcg not recommended for potential masking of vitamin B12 deficiency*

Zinc		
Risk factors for deficiency	Preexisting deficiency, malabsorptive surgery, avoidance of meat, high phytate or fiber diet, high use of antacids	
Serum marker(s)	↓ Plasma, serum, RBC, or urinary zinc	
Physical signs and symptoms	Skin lesions, poor wound healing, hair loss, taste changes, infertility, rash or acne	
Oral repletion (per day unless indicated)	**Initially:** 220 mg zinc sulfate (50 mg elemental)	**If needed progress to:** 60 mg elemental BID *Note: doses less than 30 mg may be better tolerated* *Note: recommendations based on case reports*
Copper		
Risk factors for deficiency	Malabsorption, high use of antacids, long-term use of high dose zinc supplement (more than 40 mg/d) (or zinc lozenge)	
Serum marker(s)	↓ Serum copper or ceruloplasmin	
Physical signs and symptoms	Unsteady gait, tingling in hands/feet, poor wound healing, hyperpigmentation of skin, hair, or nails	
Oral repletion (per day unless indicated)	Mild to moderate 3 to 8 mg from copper gluconate or sulfate Severe IV 2 to 4 mg six times each days	

BOX D.2 Nutrition-Related Laboratory Assessment and Related Interventions After Metabolic and Bariatric Surgery: Metabolic Bone Disorders[2-8]

Vitamin D

Risk factors for deficiency	Preexisting deficiency, malabsorption, obesity, insufficient supplementation	
Serum marker(s)	↓ 25-hydroxyvitamin D Less than 20 ng/mL (deficient); 20 to 30 ng/mL (insufficient) ↑ Alkaline phosphatase, intact parathyroid hormone, osteocalcin, N-telopeptide	
Physical signs and symptoms	Typically asymptomatic Depression, muscle pain, involuntary muscle movements, osteoporosis	
Oral repletion (per day unless indicated)	**Insufficiency:** Vitamin D3: 75 to 150 mcg (3,000 to 6,000 IU) or Vitamin D2: 1,250 mcg (50,000 IU) one to three times weekly for to 12 weeks	**Deficiency:** 50,000 to 150,000 IU/d or calcitriol 0.25 to 0.5 mcg/d

Calcium

Risk factors for deficiency	Preexisting deficiency, malabsorptive surgery, low serum vitamin D, alcoholism, insufficient or inappropriate timing of supplementation
Serum marker(s)	↓ Ionized calcium or dual energy x-ray absorptiometry scan findings suggest low bone density ↑ Alkaline phosphatase, intact parathyroid hormone (Serum calcium should always be within normal limits in absence of kidney disease)
Physical signs and symptoms	Typically asymptomatic May have bone pain or weakness or leg cramping
Oral repletion (per day unless indicated)	Biliopancreatic diversion with duodenal switch (BPD/DS): 1,800 to 2,400 mg Adjustable gastric band, sleeve gastrectomy, Roux-en-Y gastric bypass (RYGB): 1,200 to 1,500 mg *Note: Ensure serum vitamin D levels adequate* *Note: Bisphosphonates if T score less than 2.5*

BOX D.2 Nutrition-Related Laboratory Assessment and Related Interventions After Metabolic and Bariatric Surgery: Metabolic Bone Disorders[2-8] (cont.)

Vitamin K

Risk factors for deficiency	Long-limb RYGB, BPD/DS, insufficient micelle production, high-intake vitamins A and E, warfarin use, alcoholism, irritable bowel syndrome	
Serum marker(s)	↓ Plasma vitamin K ↑ Des-gamma-carboxy prothrombin ↑ Proteins induced by vitamin K absence (des gamma-carboxyprothrombin); Prothrombin time/international normalized ratio may be used but not specific or sensitive to vitamin K	
Physical signs and symptoms	Easy bruising, bleeding gums, delayed blood clotting, heavy menstrual bleeding or nose bleeds	
Oral repletion (per day unless indicated)	300 mcg	
	Acute malabsorption	**Chronic malabsorption**
	parenteral dose of 10 mg	either 1 to 2 mg or 1 to 2 mg/wk parenterally

Magnesium

Risk factors for deficiency	Inadequate intake, alcoholism, chronic diarrhea, chronic diuretic use
Serum marker(s)	↓ Serum or urinary magnesium
Physical signs and symptoms	Muscle contractions, pain, spasms, osteoporosis
Oral repletion (per day unless indicated)	No established guideline *Note: Prevention dose in nonbariatric population typically 300 to 400 mg/d* *Note: If serum mg is less than 1.5 mEq/L intravenous repletion indicated*

Appendixes

BOX D.3 Nutrition-Related Laboratory Assessment and Related Interventions After Metabolic and Bariatric Surgery: Neurologic Disorders[2-8]

Thiamin (vitamin B1)

Risk factors for deficiency	Preexisting deficiency, rapid weight loss, recurrent vomiting, intravenous (IV) glucose infusion without vitamin B1 supplementation, alcoholism, high intake of carbohydrates, antibiotics and oral contraceptives may decrease serum levels
Serum marker(s)	↓ Whole blood thiamin (thiamine pyrophosphate), erythrocyte transketolase activity ↑ Pyruvate
Physical signs and symptoms	Vomiting, numbness, tingling in extremities, gait ataxia, confusion "Dry" beriberi: convulsions, muscle weakness, pain of lower/upper extremities, brisk tendon reflexes "Wet" beriberi: tachycardia or bradycardia, lactic acidosis, dyspnea Wernicke encephalopathy: ophthalmoplegia, ataxia, confusion, hallucinations, psychosis
Oral repletion (per day unless indicated)	100 mg two to three times per day dependent on severity, until symptoms resolve or IV therapy: 200 mg, three times per day to 500 mg daily to two times per day for 3 to 5 days followed by 250 mg/d for 3 to 5 days or until symptoms resolve or Intramuscular injection therapy: 250 mg once daily for 3 to 5 days or 100 to 250 mg monthly

Appendixes

BOX D.4 Nutrition-Related Laboratory Assessment and Related Interventions After Metabolic and Bariatric Surgery: Additional Fat-Soluble Vitamins[2-8]

Vitamin A

Risk factors for deficiency	Preexisting deficiency, malabsorptive surgery, insufficient supplementation	
Serum marker(s)	↓ Plasma retinol, retinol-binding protein (RBP) (Evaluate with c-reactive protein status; RBP is an acute-phase reactant)	
Physical signs and symptoms	Loss of nocturnal vision, Bitot spots, lack of tear production, itchy dry hair, decreased immunity, poor wound healing	
Oral repletion (per day unless indicated)	**Without corneal changes** 6,000 to 7,500 mcg (10,000 to 25,000 IU) (until clinical improvement)	**With corneal changes (keratinization, ulceration, or necrosis)** (50,000 to 100,000 IU) intramuscular injection (IM) x 3 days followed by 15,000 mcg (50,000 IU) IM x 2 weeks
	Note: Risk of vitamin A toxicity occurs if daily intake higher than 100,000 IU for more than 6 months; toxicity is only of concern with ingestion of preformed (retinol) sources, no toxicity risk associated with β carotene or other provitamin A sources	

Vitamin E

Risk factors for deficiency	Biliopancreatic diversion with duodenal switch (to a minimal degree)
Serum marker(s)	↓ Plasma alpha tocopherol
Physical signs and symptoms	Hyporeflexia/weakness, gait ataxia, unexplained anemia
Oral repletion (per day unless indicated)	Optimal treatment dose currently not established *Note: 45 to 180 mg (100 to 400 IU) (antioxidant potential)*

Appendixes

References

1. Fox W, Borgert A, Rasmussen C, et al. Long-term micronutrient surveillance after gastric bypass surgery in an integrated healthcare system. *Surg Obes Relat Dis.* 2019;15(3):389-395. doi:10.1016/j.soard.2018.12.029
2. Parrott J, Frank L, Rabena R, et al. American Society for Metabolic and Bariatric Surgery Integrated Health Nutritional Guidelines for the Surgical Weight Loss Patient—2016 update: micronutrients. *Surg Obes Relat Dis.* 2016;12:955-959. doi:10.1016/j.soard.2016.12.018
3. Aills L, Blankenship J, Buffington C, Furtado M, Parrott J. ASMBS allied health nutritional guidelines for the surgical weight loss patient. *Surg Obes Relat Dis.* 2008;4:S73-S108. doi:10.1016/j.soard.2008.03.002
4. Mechanick JI, Youdim A, Jones DB, et al. Clinical practice guidelines for the perioperative nutritional, metabolic, and nonsurgical support of the bariatric surgery patient—2013 update: cosponsored by American Association of Clinical Endocrinologists, the Obesity Society, and American Society for Metabolic & Bariatric Surgery. *Obesity (Silver Spring).* 2013;21 suppl 1(01):S1-S27. doi:10.1002/oby.20461
5. Stein J, Stier C, Raab H, Weiner R. Review article: the nutritional and pharmacological consequences of obesity surgery. *Al Pharm Ther.* 2014;40:582-609. doi:10.1111/apt.12872
6. Mechanick JI, Apovian C, Brethaur S, et al. Clinical practice guidelines for the perioperative nutrition, metabolic, and nonsurgical support of patients undergoing bariatric procedures—2019 update: cosponsored by American Association of Clinical Endocrinologists/American College of Endocrinology, the Obesity Society, American Society for Metabolic & Bariatric Surgery, Obesity Medicine Association, and American Society of Anesthesiologists. *Surg Obes Relat Dis.* 2020;16(2):175-247. doi:10.4158/GL-2019-0406
7. Bays HE, Jones PH, Jacobson TA, et al. Lipids and bariatric procedures parts 1 & 2: Scientific statement from the National Lipid Association, ASMBS, OMA: executive summary. *J Clin Lipid.* 2016;10:15-32. doi:10.1016/j.jacl.2015.12.003
8. Via MA, Mechanick JI. Nutritional and micronutrient care of bariatric surgery patients: current evidence update. *Curr Obes Rep.* 2017;6:286-296. doi:10.1007/s13679-017-0271-x
9. Raymond T, Morrow K. *Krause and Mahan's food and the nutrition care process.* 15th ed. Elsevier; 2021.

APPENDIX E

Sample Nutrition Care Tools

Nutrition Care Process Documentation Tools

Figure E.1 presents a form to help the registered dietitian nutritionist (RDN) use the Nutrition Care Process (NCP) to document the assessment of a candidate for metabolic and bariatric surgery (MBS).[1] Figures E.2 and E.3 are questionnaires used during the nutrition assessment of patients in the early postoperative period (0 to 3 months post–bariatric surgery). Figure E.4 is an NCP documentation tool that RDNs can use in follow-up visits more than 6 months after MBS.

FIGURE E.1 Documentation of the initial nutrition evaluation for adult candidates for metabolic and bariatric surgery

I. Assessment

1. Reason for referral: ____________
2. Anthropometric measurements: ____________
   Weight: ____________
   Height: ____________
   BMI: ____________
3. Patient goals and expectations: ____________
   Patient's stated weight goal: ____________
   Reasons patient wants to lose weight: ____________
   Patient's expectations regarding treatment: ____________
4. Medical diagnosis/problems: ____________
5. Medications: ____________
6. Abnormal nutrition-related laboratory values (if available): ____________
7. Weight history (inquire about triggers to weight gain): ____________
   Onset of obesity (circle one): ____________
   Childhood Adolescence Adulthood
   Chronology of weight gain: ____________
   Lowest adult weight: ________ Highest adult weight: ________
   Family history of obesity: ____________
   Possible triggers to weight gain
   Life events that may have led to weight gain: ____________
   Weight-promoting medications[a]: ____________
   - ☐ Postpartum weight retention
   - ☐ Menopause
   - ☐ Smoking cessation
   - ☐ Hours of sleep per night: ____________
   - ☐ Work schedule: Shift worker?

[a]The registered dietitian nutritionist should be aware of types of medications that affect weight loss.

8. Previous weight loss efforts[b]: ______
   Prior bariatric surgery: Y/N
   Commercial programs: Y/N
   Visits with a registered dietitian nutritionist: Y/N
   Medical programs (including weight loss medications): Y/N
   Self-directed diets: Y/N
9. Current intake: ______
   Who shops and prepares food at home? ______
   ______
   Diet recall:
   Wakes: ______
   Breakfast: ______
   Snack: ______
   Lunch: ______
   Snack: ______
   Dinner: ______
   Snack: ______
   Food allergies/intolerances: ______
   Foods avoided for other reasons (eg, religious reasons):
   ______
   Vitamin/mineral supplements: ______
   ______
10. Patterns/habits: ______
    Feeling after meals: ______
    Comfortable Stuffed Can eat more
    Skips meals: Y/N
    Unplanned snacking: Y/N
    If yes, what times of day?
    Wakes during the night to eat: Y/N
    Sometimes feels "out of control" when eating: Y/N

[b]The letter of medical necessity required by all insurance providers must include patient's previous, failed attempts at weight loss and maintenance.

Nutrition quality: ___

Poor: (**a**) does not eat fruits or vegetables on a daily basis; (**b**) never eats fruits; (**c**) never eats vegetables; (**d**) consumes high amounts of processed foods; (**e**) high daily intake of empty-calorie foods (sweets, fatty/salty foods)

Good: (**a**) eats some fruits and/or vegetables daily; (**b**) "tries" to eat healthy—whole wheat bread; (**c**) moderate to high intake of empty-calorie foods (sweets, salty/fatty foods)

Excellent: (**a**) daily intake of fruits and vegetables; (**b**) eats whole grains, lean meats, low-fat meals.

Consumption of high-calorie beverages: Y/N

If yes, what kind: ___

Juice Soda Whole milk Alcohol

Eating out: Note how often per day/week/month

Fast-food restaurants: ___

Take-out or delivery: ___

Restaurants: ___

11. Physical activity pattern: ___

Work-related activity: ___

Sedentary Moderate Heavy

Time spent in sedentary activities per day (computer, TV, etc.):

___

Planned exercise (type): ___

Time spent in planned exercise: ___

If patient does not exercise, are there specific barriers to exercise?

___

II. Nutrition Diagnosis[c]

1. Intake: ___

- ☐ Excessive energy intake
- ☐ Excessive fluid intake
- ☐ Excessive alcohol intake
- ☐ Excessive fat intake
- ☐ Other: ___

[c] Documentation of each nutrition diagnosis should be in the form of a PES (problem, etiology, signs and symptoms) statement.

2. Clinical: ______

- ☐ Overweight/obesity
- ☐ Unintended weight gain
- ☐ Other: ______

3. Behavioral-Environmental: ______

- ☐ Food- and nutrition-related knowledge deficit
- ☐ Not ready for diet/lifestyle change
- ☐ Disordered eating pattern
- ☐ Undesirable food choices
- ☐ Physical inactivity
- ☐ Inability to manage self-care
- ☐ Other: ______

III. Nutrition Intervention

1. Food and/or Nutrient Delivery: Meals and snacks
   Decreased energy diet
   Other: ______
2. Coordination of Nutrition Care by Nutrition Professional (PCP, surgeon, psychologist/other mental health provider, surgical multidisciplinary care team)
   Other: ______

IV. RDN Recommendations

1. Does the registered dietitian nutritionist have any nutrition/behavioral or other concerns regarding consideration of bariatric surgery? Y/N
2. If so, list and/or describe:______
3. Does the registered dietitian nutritionist support the decision for bariatric surgery? Y/N

FIGURE E.2 Patient questionnaire for the first nutrition visit 2 weeks after metabolic and bariatric surgery (advancing the diet to semisolid textures)

Today's date: ______________________________

Date of surgery: ______________________________

Today's weight: ______________________________

Type of surgical procedure: ______________________________

1. Did you have complications after bariatric surgery that affected your ability to follow the diet guidelines you were given?
   No Yes
2. If yes, explain: ______________________________
3. List any medications you are currently taking: ______________________________
4. Check any of the following that you are experiencing:
   - ☐ Vomiting episodes
   - ☐ Dumping syndrome
   - ☐ Diarrhea
   - ☐ Constipation
   - ☐ Nausea episodes
5. For each box checked in Question 4, please list the triggers or causes:
   ____
   ____
6. How many ounces or servings of "full" liquid do you consume every day (this includes protein shakes, milk, yogurt, etc)? ______________________________
   ____
7. If you were unable to consume the minimum recommended amount of full liquid, explain why. ______________________________
   ____
   ____
8. How many ounces or glasses of "clear" liquid (water and other calorie-free, noncarbonated liquids) have you been consuming every day?
   ____

9. Have you started taking a multivitamin?

   No Yes (list type) ______________________________

10. Have you started taking a calcium supplement?

    No Yes (list type) ______________________________

11. Have you started taking your B12 vitamin?

    No Yes

12. Have you started taking your vitamin D supplement?

    No Yes

13. Do you have a schedule of all of your nutrition follow-up groups or appointments?

    No Yes

FIGURE E.3 Assessment information to include in 12-week nutrition visit documentation

Today's date: ______

1. Medical diagnosis: ______
2. Medications: ______
3. Surgery date: ______
4. Surgery procedure: ______
5. Nutrition-related laboratory values: ______
6. Patient experiences:
   - ☐ Nausea/vomiting
   - ☐ Dumping syndrome
   - ☐ Chronic diarrhea
   - ☐ Constipation

   Other: ______
7. Other food/eating-related problems/concerns: ______
8. Reported intake:

   Number of meals/day: ______

   Number of snacks/day: ______

   Reported intake of clear liquids consumed/day: ______

   Patient reports mindless eating/snacking: Y/N

   Reported intake of protein at each meal: ______

   Reported intake of fruits daily: ______

   Reported intake of vegetables daily: ______

   Is patient drinking liquids with meals? Y/N

   Is patient avoiding carbonated beverages? Y/N

   Is patient drinking alcoholic beverages? Y/N

9. Nutritional supplementation:

   Is patient taking recommended multivitamin with iron daily? Y/N

   Is patient taking recommended calcium supplement? Y/N

   What type of calcium? ______________________________

   Is patient taking calcium in divided doses? Y/N

   How many doses a day? ______________________________

   Is patient taking vitamin D supplement? Y/N

   Amount: ______________________________

   Is patient taking supplemental vitamin B12? Y/N

   Is patient taking other prescription or over-the-counter supplements? Y/N
   List types: ______________________________

10. Foods/beverages not tolerated: ______________________________
11. Does patient feel deprived? Y/N
12. Does patient feel restricted? Y/N
13. Does patient have problems with adapting to new eating habits/behaviors? Y/N
14. Physical activity: ______________________________

    ____

15. Does patient verbalize need for additional psychological or nutrition support? Y/N

FIGURE E.4 Documentation of follow-up nutrition visits (6 months or more after metabolic and bariatric surgery)

I. Assessment

1. Problems: ______
2. Medications: ______
3. Weight: ______
4. BMI: ______
5. Surgery date: ______
6. Surgery procedure: ______
7. Weight change since surgery: ______
8. Abnormal nutrition-related laboratory data: ______
   ______
9. Patient complications:
   - ☐ Nausea/vomiting
   - ☐ Dumping syndrome
   - ☐ Chronic diarrhea
   - ☐ Constipation
10. Other food/eating-related problems: ______
11. Eating habits/tolerances:
    Does patient experience physical hunger? Y/N
    Foods not tolerated: ______
    ______
12. Diet assessment:
    Number of meals/day: ______
    Number of snacks/day: ______
    Adequacy of intake:
    Adequate protein intake: Y/N
    Eats fruits daily: Y/N
    Eats vegetables daily: Y/N
    Total ounces of fluid per day: ______

Is patient waiting 30 minutes after eating before drinking? Y/N

Does patient drink alcohol? Y/N

If yes, how much per day/week/month? ______________________

13. Nutritional supplementation:

Daily multivitamin with iron: Y/N

Supplemental calcium: Y/N Amount: ______________________

Supplemental vitamin B12: Y/N

Prescribed or other supplements: Y/N

List types and amounts: ______________________

____

14. Exercise/Activity: Y/N

If yes, what type of exercise and duration? ______________________

If no, what is limiting activity? ______________________

____

II. Nutrition Diagnosis[a]

1. Intake:

a. Excessive energy intake

b. Excessive fat intake

c. Inconsistent carbohydrate intake

d. Inadequate carbohydrate intake

e. Excessive oral intake

f. Excessive alcohol intake

g. Intake of types of fats inconsistent with needs (specify)

h. Intake of types of carbohydrate inconsistent with needs (specify)

i. Inadequate fiber intake

j. Inadequate fluid intake

k. Excessive fluid intake

l. Other: ______________________

[a]Selected examples of potential nutrition diagnoses. Documentation of each nutrition diagnosis should be in the form of a PES (problem, etiology, signs and symptoms) statement.

2. Clinical:
   a. Overweight/obesity
   b. Unintended weight gain
   c. Other: ______________________
3. Behavioral/Environmental:
   a. Food- and nutrition-related knowledge deficit
   b. Not ready for diet/lifestyle change
   c. Self monitoring deficit
   d. Disordered eating pattern
   e. Undesirable food choices
   f. Limited adherence to nutrition-related recommendations
   g. Physical inactivity
   h. Poor nutrition quality of life
   i. Inability to manage self care
   j. Other: ______________________

III. Nutrition Intervention

Selected interventions:

1. Food and/or Nutrient Delivery:
   a. Meals and snacks:
   - Modify composition of meals/snacks
   - Diets modified for specific foods or ingredients
   - Other: ______________________
2. Nutrition-related medication management
   a. Management of nutrition-related prescription medication
   b. Management of nutrition-related over-the-counter (OTC) medication
3. Coordination of Nutrition Care by a Nutrition Professional
4. Nutrition Education:
   a. Content-related nutrition education
   b. Education on nutrition's influence on health
   c. Physical activity guidance

d. Nutrition-related laboratory result interpretation

e. Nutrition-related skill education

f. Technical nutrition education

5. Nutrition Counseling:

a. Nutrition counseling based on cognitive behavioral theory approach

b. Nutrition counseling based on motivational interviewing strategy

c. Nutrition counseling based on self monitoring strategy

d. Nutrition counseling based on stress management strategy

IV. Nutrition Monitoring and Evaluation

Outcome Indicators

The following are examples, not an all-inclusive list. Registered dietitian nutritionists are encouraged to use the outcome indicators for each nutrition intervention as appropriate.

1. Food- and Nutrition-Related History:

a. Total fluid estimated intake in 24 hours

b. Total energy estimated intake in 24 hours

c. Total fat estimated intake in 24 hours

d. Estimated amount of food

e. Knowledge/Beliefs/Attitudes

- Nutrition knowledge of supportive individuals
- Conflict with personal/family value system
- Distorted body image

f. Type of food/meals

g. Meal/snack pattern

h. Self reported nutrition adherence score

i. Physical activity:

- Consistency
- Frequency
- Duration
- Intensity
- Strength

2. Nutrition-Focused Physical Findings:
   a. Digestive system (eg, reduction or elimination of reports of diarrhea)
3. Anthropometric Measurements:
   a. Body mass index (BMI)
   b. Measured weight
   c. Weight change
4. Biochemical Data, Medical Tests, and Procedures:
   a. Urine volume
   b. Urine color

Monitoring and Evaluation Summary: ______________________

____

____

Assessment of Adjustable Gastric Band Patient's Hunger/Need for Fill

The form in Figure E.5 is used in conjunction with the nutrition assessment to determine whether an adjustable gastric banding patient needs a fill at the time of a nutrition follow-up visit. The questionnaires in Figures E.3 or E.4 may be used with this form.

FIGURE E.5 Adjustable gastric banding (AGB) hunger survey

This survey will help determine whether a "fill" is needed.

Today's date: ______________________

Today's weight: ______________________

Date of last fill: ______________________

Weight at last fill: ______________________

The following questions ask about experiences with hunger and fullness. Your feelings may vary from day to day or from meal to meal. Answer questions about how you feel "on average."

Hunger

In the following questions, hunger is defined as a physical feeling in the body.

1. Check all that describe your feelings of hunger.
   - ☐ Feeling of emptiness in your body
   - ☐ Fatigue
   - ☐ General feeling of needing to eat or drink
   - ☐ Physical sensations in your stomach (such as grumbling or discomfort)
   - ☐ Abdominal pain
   - ☐ Light-headedness
   - ☐ Irritability
   - ☐ Other: ______________________
   - ☐ I don't know what hunger feels like.
   - ☐ I never experience hunger.
2. Since your last fill, how often have you experienced hunger?
   - ☐ Never
   - ☐ Every few days
   - ☐ Almost every day
   - ☐ 1-2 times a day
   - ☐ Several times a day
   - ☐ Always hungry

3. Since your last **fill**, how strong have your feelings of hunger typically been?
   - ☐ Unable to eat
   - ☐ Not hungry
   - ☐ Slightly hungry
   - ☐ Moderately hungry
   - ☐ Very hungry
   - ☐ Absolutely "starving"

Fullness

The following questions address feelings of fullness. These feelings may include a general **physical** feeling that you have had enough to eat.

1. Since your last **fill,** how full do you feel, in general, after you finish a snack or meal?
   - ☐ Slightly hungry
   - ☐ Moderately hungry
   - ☐ Totally empty
   - ☐ Not at all full
   - ☐ Slightly full
   - ☐ Moderately full
   - ☐ Very full
   - ☐ Absolutely "stuffed"
2. Since your last **fill**, how long after you start eating do you typically notice feelings of fullness?
   - ☐ 0-5 minutes
   - ☐ 6-10 minutes
   - ☐ 11-15 minutes
   - ☐ 16-20 minutes
   - ☐ 20-30 minutes
   - ☐ More than 30 minutes

3. Since your last **fill**, how long after feeling full do you generally become physically hungry again?
   - ☐ 0-14 minutes
   - ☐ 15-30 minutes
   - ☐ 30 minutes-1 hour
   - ☐ 1-3 hours
   - ☐ More than 3 hours
   - ☐ I never feel hungry

Reference

1. Academy of Nutrition and Dietetics. Nutrition Terminology Reference Manual (eNCPT): dietetics language for nutrition care. Accessed June 5, 2021. http://ncpt.webauthor.com

APPENDIX F

Postoperative Complications and Symptom Management*

Patients should go to the nearest emergency department and contact their medical team if they experience any of the following:

- temperature higher than 100.5 ° F
- an incision that opens or becomes red, swollen, or tender
- nausea, vomiting, or shortness of breath
- vomiting of blood
- chest pain or shortness of breath not relieved by rest
- pain or swelling of the legs
- black or bloody stool

* Adapted with permission from practice documents developed by Kellene A. Isom, PhD, MS, RD, CAGS

Complications of the Roux-en-Y Gastric Bypass and Sleeve Gastrectomy

Stricture

The outlet between the stomach (gastric pouch) and the intestine (jejunum), called the anastomosis, can narrow after Roux-en-Y gastric bypass (RYGB) surgery, thus restricting the passage of food. Symptoms of a stricture include:

- abdominal pain,
- vomiting, and
- decreased oral intake.

Narrowing of the gastric sleeve can occur after sleeve gastrectomy (SG) surgery, thus restricting the passage of food. Stricture may result in food intolerance and vomiting after eating.[1]

Strictures may occur in 2.3% of SG patients and are more likely to occur within 8 weeks after surgery. Strictures in RYGB patients can occur at any time. They range in occurrence from 4.7% to 16% of patients. Anastomotic strictures are usually first managed with endoscopic balloon dilation and consecutive endoscopic dilations or revisional surgery if needed.[2]

Wound Infection

Wound infections are uncommon following laparoscopic procedures; however, if a patient experiences any wound infection within the first few weeks after surgery, they should do the following:

- Call the medical team immediately.
- Make sure the patient is getting adequate protein to help with healing.
- Drink plenty of fluids.
- Take multivitamins daily.

Signs of a wound infection include, yellow, yellow-green, or foul-smelling discharge, redness, swelling, pain around the wound, or fever.

For revisions that convert the adjustable gastric band (AGB) to the RYGB, wound infections are the most common complication, with a 7% occurrence.[2]

Leg Cramps

If the patient experiences leg cramps within the first few weeks after surgery, they should do the following:

- Call the medical team immediately if cramps persist or present with swelling. The patient should be evaluated for potential blood clot.
- Eat a well-balanced diet (include potassium-rich foods, such as yogurt, white beans, tuna, steamed/soft broccoli, bananas, and milk).
- Take supplements as directed.
- Stay physically active. Patients should resume walking immediately after surgery, generally starting the day of surgery, as able.
- Drink plenty of fluids.

Vomiting

If the patient vomits bright red or dark brown liquid, they should contact the medical team immediately. The medical team may advise the patient to return to a clear liquid diet and seek to rule out infection (eg, *Clostridium difficile*), gastrointestinal bleed, obstruction, or ileus. In the case of intractable vomiting, intravenous (IV) thiamin should be given to prevent Wernicke encephalopathy. See Appendix D for more information about thiamin/vitamin Bl deficiency.

Regurgitation

If the patient regurgitates chewed (without blood) food shortly after eating, they may not be chewing food thoroughly or ate too quickly. The patient may be advised to do the following:

- Return to the full liquid diet for 1 to 2 days.
- Return to an earlier diet stage that is more tolerable, such as protein drinks if the patient is currently on semisolids or semisolids if the patient is currently on soft textures.
- Take small, dime-size bites and chew foods thoroughly; eat slowly.
- Avoid overeating; eat mindfully; stop when comfortable.
- Make sure foods are moist (particularly meats).
- Avoid eating and drinking at the same time; wait 30 minutes after eating before drinking.

Dehydration

If the patient experiences dizziness, nausea, dark urine, headaches, or light-headedness within the first few weeks after surgery, they should do the following:

- Confirm proper medication changes. Diuretic agents must be discontinued or halved prior to discharge. Present immediately to the emergency department or speak to their metabolic and bariatric providers for IV hydration.
- Metabolic and bariatric surgery (MBS) providers may recommend a banana bag or IV thiamin along with IV hydration to prevent potential Wernicke encephalopathy. Normal saline (vs a glucose containing solution) is recommended.
- Drink plenty of water and other low-calorie fluids with electrolytes (eg, Smart Water, Propel, G2, Gatorade Zero, and Powerade Zero) to prevent dehydration.
- Drink regular bouillon/broth.

Obstruction

An obstruction can be a severe, early postoperative complication after RYGB and biliopancreatic diversion with duodenal switch (BPD/DS) surgery. Luckily it is rare, only occurring in 0% to 5% of patients. Similar to other types of bowel obstruction, patients may present with the following symptoms[2]:

- abdominal pain
- vomiting
- nausea
- minimal bowel function
- postoperative edema or hematoma involving the gastrojejunal (G-J) or jejunojejunal (J-J) anastomosis, which is most indicative of an early obstruction

Leak

A leak between the connections of the stomach (gastric pouch) and intestine can occur after RYGB and BPD/DS surgery. A leak along the staple line of the gastric sleeve can also occur after SG surgery. The pouch can be tested in the operating room for leaks, but leaks may still occur immediately postoperatively. Signs of a leak include a rapid heartbeat, severe abdominal pain, leukocytosis, and fever.[1,2] Increased risk factors for patients who develop leaks after RYGB include an open operative technique, revision surgery, age older than 50 years, male sex, congestive heart failure, chronic renal failure, and chronic lung disease. The rate of leaks after RYGB surgery range from 0.7% to 5% of patients. The lower rates occur with more modern-day laparoscopic techniques. A proximal, difficult-to-fix leak in the early postoperative period after the SG is rare but serious (4.9% of cases), while long-term management of leaks as a complication have been reported to occur in 2.4% of patients.[2]

Ulcers

Ulcers can cause bleeding at any time after RYGB and BPD/DS surgery. Ulcers can be marginal, anastomotic, or a gastric pouch ulceration. Patients may present with abdominal pain, blood in their vomit or stool. There is a 4% incidence for marginal ulcers, and they are diagnosed via endoscopy on the G-J anastomosis, proximal jejunal limb adjacent to the anastomosis, and gastric pouch. Treatment includes smoking and alcohol cessation, discontinuation of ulcerogenic medications (such as non-steroidal anti-inflammatories [NSAIDs], and the use of a proton pump inhibitor alone or combined with sucralfate.[2]

Complications of Adjustable Gastric Banding

Band Erosion

The band may erode through the stomach wall in 2.8% of patients. Erosion rarely leads to free perforation or sepsis. Erosion is thought to be due to operative injury to the gastric wall or a band that is too tight and overinflated. Band erosion is best diagnosed by endoscopy and treated by surgical removal of the band.[1-4]

Esophageal Dilation

Esophageal dilation is a serious condition, with a risk of esophageal motility dysfunction. It can occur in 5% to 71% of patients. The etiology is likely to be overinflation of the band.[2] Esophageal dilatation may lead to backup of consumed food in the distal esophagus. The condition is diagnosed by fluoroscopic x-ray of the upper gastrointestinal tract (UGI). The condition may be asymptomatic; yearly testing is suggested. Esophageal dilatation may require surgical removal of the band.[1-4]

Band Prolapse or Band Slippage

Slippage occurs when the stomach above or below the band slips or prolapses through the band. This narrows the opening between the pouch and the lower stomach. Prolapse results in obstruction of the pouch or herniation of the fundus. Prolapse may be due to poor fixation of the band or dietary noncompliance. It can occur in 4% to 12.5% of patients.[2] Band prolapse is diagnosed by UGI. The condition may resolve with band deflation.[1-4]

Signs and symptoms of prolapse include abdominal pain, nausea/vomiting, gastroesophageal reflux, dysphagia (difficulty swallowing liquids), night cough, chest pain or pressure, and gastric obstruction. Treatment for prolapse involves the following[1-4]:

- saline removal from band to increase the stoma
- diet texture regression to liquids and then progression to semisolids
- allowing the stomach to slip back down
- review of eating style changes
- new operation to secure the band

Long-Term Micronutrient Deficiencies After Metabolic and Bariatric Surgery

See Appendixes C and D.

References

1. Mechanick JI, Kushner RF, Sugerman HJ, et al. Executive summary of the recommendations of the American Association of Clinical Endocrinologists, the Obesity Society, and American Society for Metabolic and Bariatric Surgery medical guidelines for clinical practice for the perioperative nutritional, metabolic, and nonsurgical support of the bariatric surgery patient. *Endocr Pract.* 2008;14:318-336. doi:10.1002/oby.20461
2. Ma IT, Madura II JA. Gastrointestinal complications after bariatric surgery. *Gastroenterol Hepatol (N.Y.).* 2015;11(8):526-535.
3. Lattuada E, Zappa MA, Mozzi E, et al. Band erosion following gastric banding: how to treat it. *Obes Surg.* 2007;17:329-333. doi:10.1007/s11695-007-9060-z
4. Chevallier JM, Zinzindohoué F, Douard R, et al. Complications after laparoscopic adjustable gastric banding for morbid obesity: experience with 1,000 patients over 7 years. *Obes Surg.* 2004;14:407-414. doi:10.1381/096089204322917954

APPENDIX G

Nutrition Troubleshooting Guide for the Metabolic and Bariatric Surgery Patient

Note: The problems presented here may have nutritional implications. Advise all patients to call their surgeon or primary care physician or to go directly to an emergency department if any of the problems are not related to diet.

Constipation

Constipation may occur within the first few weeks after surgery because fiber intake is low. In addition, potential etiologies of the occurrence of constipation at any time point after metabolic and bariatric surgery (MBS) include the following:

- narcotic usage

- decreased fluid intake
- a low-fiber diet
- calcium supplementation
- iron supplementation, particularly if the therapeutic dosage is greater than the Recommended Dietary Allowance[1]
- certain types of iron salts, such as ferrous sulfate
- use of protein pump inhibitors or other acid-reducing medications
- limited activity

When a patient has constipation, fluid and fiber intake and physical activity level should be assessed. If fluid and fiber intake are inadequate, efforts should be made to increase them. In addition, the patient should take the lowest dosage of iron needed. Supplemental fiber is an option if dietary fiber is not meeting the patient's fiber needs.

Patients whose constipation continues for an extended period of time should consult with their surgeon or primary care physician (PCP). If increased fluid and fiber intake do not help alleviate constipation, patients may need to take a stool softener or laxative. A lack of bowel movements for 3 to 4 days warrants the use of a stool softener or laxative. Some registered dietitian nutritionists will use preventive measures soon after surgery. Since constipation can lead to abdominal pain, which may be confused for surgical pain, prevention may help reduce this.

Advise patients to do the following:

- Stay physically active.
- Drink plenty of water (48 to 64 oz/d).
- Increase soluble and insoluble fiber intake with fruits, vegetables, and whole grains. Some patients may experience relief with soluble vs insoluble fiber and vice versa.
    - When consuming semisolid and soft-textured foods, consumption of soft fruits and vegetables is encouraged.
    - When consuming regular textures, consumption of high-fiber cereals can help patients increase fiber intake.

Dumping Syndrome

Dumping syndrome is reported in about 40% of postoperative Roux-en-Y gastric bypass (RYGB) patients.[2] This condition is due to the lack of a pyloric sphincter and occurs after consumption of high-sugar and high-carbohydrate-containing foods, which create a hypertonic solution in the jejunum. This hypertonic solution leads to sudden distension of the jejunum, resulting in symptoms of early dumping syndrome (nausea, dizziness, weakness, rapid pulse, cold sweats, fatigue, cramps, and diarrhea) 10 to 30 minutes after eating.[3,4] Another potential mechanism may be the release of GI hormones, such as vasoactive agents, incretins (eg, glucagon-like peptide-1 [GLP-1]), and glucose modulators, that increase gastrointestinal (GI) motility.[2,5] Dumping does not appear to be common with the one-anastomosis gastric bypass (OAGB), potentially related to a slower absorption of sugars from longer contact of food with biliopancreatic (BP) secretions.[6]

Dumping can be diagnosed using symptoms-based questionnaires, glycemic monitoring, or an oral glucose or mixed meal tolerance test.[2] In the presence of normal blood glucose levels, dumping can be expected.[5] Questionnaires (eg, Sigstad's score, used to separate patients with dumping; Arts's dumping questionnaire, used to determine early vs late dumping) may be used.[2]

Some RYGB patients experience late dumping syndrome, which occurs 1 to 3 hours after a meal. This occurs when the rapid absorption of glucose triggers an exaggerated insulin release, causing reactive hypoglycemia.[4,7]

Sleeve gastrectomy (SG) patients may have symptoms reminiscent of dumping syndrome, but they are most likely caused by reactive hypoglycemia. The exact mechanism is still unknown.[7,8]

Box G.1 describes behaviors that can prevent dumping syndrome.[4] See Chapter 7 for recommendations on the dietary management of reactive hypoglycemia.

At this time, there is insufficient evidence to support the use of dietary supplements in the treatment of dumping. Pharmacologic intervention may include acarbose (an alpha-glucosidase hydrolase inhibitor that slows carbohydrate digestion in the small intestine but may only be

BOX G.1 Tips to Prevent Dumping Syndrome[5,6]

Consume foods and beverages containing a *hypotonic* solution.

Avoid *hypertonic* solutions, such as juice, soda, frosting, and other concentrated sweets and foods with added sugar.

Limit food choices to less than 20 to 25 g *total* sugar per serving.

Avoid *added* sugars, including sucrose, honey, and high-fructose corn syrup.

Do not avoid natural sugars, such as those in dairy products and fruit.

Pair high fiber/low glycemic carbohydrate-based foods with a protein or fat.

Reduce the amount of food consumed at each meal

Avoid consuming liquids with meals and chew food thoroughly.

effective for late dumping) and somatostatin analogues (target delayed gastric emptying, delaying transit through the small intestine, inhibiting the release of gastrointestinal (GI) hormones, and inhibiting insulin secretion and postprandial vasodilation). See Chapter 7 and Box 7.3 on page 154 for more pharmacologic interventions. Other pharmacologic agents have been evaluated, but studies are small and lack supporting evidence.[2]

Diarrhea

Patients without chronic diarrhea before surgery may experience softer stools or diarrhea within the first few weeks after surgery. Adjustable gastric banding (AGB), RYGB, and SG procedures should not cause long-term diarrhea. Patients who report excessive gas and diarrhea may have lactose intolerance. Biliopancreatic diversion with duodenal switch (BPD/DS) patients may experience more frequent bowel movements, typically more than two per day;[9] they should be encouraged to avoid foods high in sugar and fat that may exacerbate diarrhea. One-anastomosis gastric bypass (OAGB) patients report an average increase of half a bowel movement per day before surgery to two per day after.[10] Drinking fluids while eating solid foods may also cause diarrhea because liquids speed up the passage of food through the GI tract.

If a patient experiences diarrhea that is not related to lactose intolerance or drinking with meals, the patient should contact the medical team immediately and return to the clear liquid diet for 1 or 2 days. Infection, dumping syndrome, small intestinal bacterial overgrowth (SIBO), and other dietary causes of diarrhea, such as the use of sugar alcohols, should be considered as possible etiologies. Approximately 40% of RYGB may experience SIBO, but without a true gold standard for diagnosing SIBO, this is hard to estimate.[11]

If diarrhea occurs within the first few weeks after surgery, advise patients to do the following:

- Limit or avoid foods with lactose or sugar alcohols.
- Seek assessment for food intolerances.
- Eat slowly and chew thoroughly.
- Avoid drinking fluids with meals.
- Avoid high-sugar, high-fat, and spicy foods.
- Limit consumption of sugar-free products that contain sugar alcohols.
- Limit food products containing inulin or chicory root, as this may cause a laxative effect for some.
- Limit intake of caffeinated beverages.
- Discuss with health care team whether a probiotic supplement with *Lactobacillus* might be helpful.[12]
- Discuss any new medications that may be causing diarrhea, for example, metformin or omeprazole.
- *Clostridium difficile* infection or SIBO may also need to be ruled out if diarrhea continues.

The latter may be considered if diarrhea occurs at any time point after MBS.

Regurgitation or Vomiting*

If patients experience regurgitation of chewed food shortly after eating, they may not be chewing food thoroughly or may be eating too quickly. Advise patients to do the following:

- Return to the full liquid diet for 1 to 2 days.
- Return to an earlier diet stage that is more tolerable. For example, if the patient is currently on regular textures, return to soft textures; if the patient is currently on soft textures, return to semisolid textures.
- Take small bites, chew foods thoroughly, and eat slowly.
- Avoid overeating; eat mindfully; stop when comfortable.
- Make sure foods are moist (particularly meats).
- Avoid eating and drinking at the same time; wait 30 minutes after eating before drinking.

Nausea

Patients may experience nausea in the first few weeks after surgery. The use of narcotics can increase nausea. In addition to management provided by the medical team, advise patients to do the following:

- Avoid overeating.
- Drink plenty of fluids (48 to 64 oz/d); nausea is often triggered when a patient is dehydrated.
- Avoid plain water; low-calorie fluids with solutes (eg, electrolytes or flavored waters) may not feel as hard on the stomach.
- Chew foods thoroughly and eat slowly.
- Avoid carbonated beverages.
- Avoid foods that are not tolerated.
- Avoid eating and drinking at the same time.

* If the following suggestions do not work or vomit is bright red or dark brown, patients should contact their medical team immediately (see Appendix F for more information).

- Avoid foods that may cause dumping syndrome (candies, cookies, cakes, sugary drinks, pastries, and sweetened breads).
- Limit or avoid foods with lactose.

The medical team may assess patients for symptoms of heartburn/gastroesophageal reflux disorder. In some cases of nausea, antiemetics may be prescribed.

Dehydration

A patient may become dehydrated as a result of inadequate fluid intake or because of fluid losses from vomiting or severe diarrhea. Signs and symptoms of dehydration include the following:

- dark urine
- fatigue
- nausea/vomiting
- dizziness upon standing (hypotension)
- headache
- extreme weight loss

If dehydration is suspected, the registered dietitian nutritionist (RDN) should assess fluid intake and, if appropriate, recommend intravenous (IV) hydration. IV solutions that contain dextrose or other sugar solutions may exacerbate thiamin deficiency. Therefore, IV hydration solutions should contain thiamin, which is utilized in the metabolism of carbohydrates. Undetected thiamin deficiency can lead to beriberi or Wernicke encephalopathy.

Patients may not consume adequate fluids because they must sip liquids and because they should not drink during or 30 minutes after a snack or meal. The RDN should encourage patients to drink clear liquids frequently, even when they do not desire them.

When patients are nauseous, they often do not tolerate fluids, which can worsen dehydration. An antiemetic may help alleviate nausea and prevent more severe dehydration.

Patients who take hypertensive medications that contain diuretics or who continue a diuretic after MBS are at higher risk for dehydration. The RDN may advise patients to follow-up frequently with their primary care physician in the early postoperative days and weeks to ensure they receive the appropriate dosages of medications to manage their blood pressure and avoid dehydration.

Stomach Bloating

If patients have stomach bloating after eating within the first few weeks after surgery, advise them to do the following:

- Avoid overeating.
- Avoid drinking fluids with meals.
- Avoid carbonated beverages.
- Stay physically active.
- Avoid sugar alcohols, inulin, or chicory root.
- Limit or avoid foods with lactose.

Lactose Intolerance

If patients are unable to tolerate dairy products within the first few weeks after surgery, advise them to do the following:

- Limit or avoid all lactose-containing products, including protein shakes.
- Try lactose-free milk.
- Try lactase enzyme tablets or drops.
- Consume dairy products that contain less lactose (eg, low-fat yogurt, hard cheeses, and kefir).

Patients who experience lactose intolerance before MBS are likely to also experience it after surgery. Some patients also report developing lactose intolerance after surgery. Many of the liquid supplements recommended for a full liquid diet contain lactose. The RDN should advise patients with lactose intolerance to consume full liquids composed of whey protein isolates, soy-based protein, or other lactose-free, protein-containing full liquids.

The RDN should counsel patients with suspected or confirmed lactose intolerance to check ingredient lists on products to determine whether they contain lactose. See Box G.2 for ingredients that should be avoided.

BOX G.2 Ingredients Containing Lactose

- Ammonium caseinate
- Artificial butter flavor
- Butter solids/fat
- Calcium caseinate
- Casein
- Caseinate
- Delactosed whey
- Demineralized whey
- Dried milk
- Dried milk solids
- Hydrolyzed casein
- Hydrolyzed milk protein
- Lactalbumin
- Lactalbumin phosphate
- Lactate
- Lactoferrin
- Lactoglobulin
- Lactose
- Magnesium caseinate
- Milk derivative
- Milk fat
- Milk protein
- Milk solids
- Opta (fat replacement)
- Potassium caseinate
- Rennet casein
- Simplesse
- Sodium caseinate
- Sour cream solids
- Sour milk solids
- Whey protein concentrate

Food Intolerances and Other Eating Problems

Food intolerances are common in the period immediately following bariatric surgery. Patients may also have altered taste and changes in food preferences. Regurgitation without nausea or true vomiting is common when patients eat or drink too much food, eat or drink too rapidly, or do not chew food thoroughly. Patients may find regular reminders to eat and drink slowly and use mindful eating exercises to be helpful.

Patients may report that food gets "stuck." They may experience this problem more often when food is poorly chewed or when eating dry meats, chicken, other dense proteins, sticky foods (eg, peanut butter), and some starches, such as bread, rice, or pasta. Patients who experience "sticking" with these foods should be advised to either avoid them or modify them so they are better tolerated.

Overall, food tolerance appears to be best in SG patients, followed by the RYGB.[13] Foods like dry, tough meat, doughy bread, fibrous fruits or vegetables, and high-sugar/high-fat foods may not be tolerated, but variances exist among individuals.

Protein Malnutrition

Risk After Metabolic and Bariatric Surgery

Protein malnutrition is uncommon in uncomplicated MBS patients but is a risk if oral intake is poor or complications occur.[14] Protein malnutrition is most likely in patients who have undergone BPD/DS procedures, as 3% to 5% of cases experience protein calorie malnutrition[15] and up to 13% of patients with distal RYGB, depending on Roux limb length.[16] Rates of malnutrition for OAGB are reported in 0.2% to 1.1% of cases[6] and 6% to 23% in single-anastomosis duodeno-ileostomy with sleeve (SADI-S)[17] but definitions of malnutrition are not consistent among studies (eg, hypoalbuminemia and loss of fat-free mass). In these patients, early occurrences of protein malnutrition have been used due to patient-related factors, such as inadequate protein intake or intolerance to protein-based foods, whereas late episodes of protein malnutrition in BPD/DS, OAGB, and certain revisional procedures may be a consequence of malabsorption.[17]

Malabsorption has not been found to be the mechanism of protein malnutrition in patients who undergo MBS procedures other than the BPD/DS and distal RYGB. In these cases, protein malnutrition is associated with concurrent issues that lead to decreased energy and protein intake, such as prolonged vomiting, diarrhea, food intolerance, alcohol or drug abuse, or a limited food budget. Some of these factors are not necessarily a result of the surgery itself.

Although MBS patients have been shown to have lower intakes of protein 1 year postoperatively when compared with their preoperative intake,[18,19] hypoalbuminemia is uncommon . Additionally, hypoalbuminemia is not an accurate criteria for the diagnosis of malnutrition.[19-20] It is uncommon for RYGB, SG, and AGB patients to develop protein malnutrition because the body can adapt to short-term periods of low protein intake, and these surgeries are not malabsorptive.[20,21]

Dizziness, Lightheadedness, or Headaches

If patients experience dizziness, lightheadedness, or headaches within the first few weeks after surgery, advise them to do the following:

- Drink plenty of water and other low-calorie fluids with electrolytes (eg, electrolyte-enhanced waters or low-calorie, electrolyte-enhanced sports beverages) to prevent dehydration.
- Add salt to foods.
- Drink regular bouillon/broth.
- Ensure adequate food intake.
- Eat on a regular schedule (about every 3 hours).
- Contact the physician or go to the emergency department to be assessed for dehydration.

- Avoid concentrated sugars and avoid drinking while eating, since light-headedness with fatigue is a symptom of dumping syndrome.
- Check with their primary care provider or MBS medical team to identify hypotension; most patients require changes in hypertension and diabetes-related medications after surgery.

Fatigue or General Weakness

If patients experience fatigue or general weakness within the first few weeks after surgery, advise them to do the following:

- Drink plenty of fluids.
- Avoid caffeine.
- Sleep on a regular schedule.
- Stay physically active.
- Ensure adequate calorie, protein, and carbohydrate (fruits/vegetables) intake and eat on a schedule.
- Take daily vitamin/mineral supplements as instructed by the health care team.

Heartburn

If patients have heartburn within the first few weeks after surgery, advise them to do the following:

- Eat every 4 hours. Avoid going long periods of time without eating.
- Avoid caffeinated beverages.
- Avoid spicy foods.
- Avoid aspirin or other nonsteroidal anti-inflammatory drugs.
- Take over-the-counter medications or prescribed medications for heartburn relief as directed. Patients are put on proton pump inhibitors post-MBS. It is important to assess their adherence with these medications.

- Avoid foods that are too hot or too cold.
- Avoid lying down for 2 hours after eating.
- Avoid alcoholic beverages.

The medical team should check whether heartburn could be an adverse effect of any medications the patient is taking.

In addition, patients may often confuse feelings of fullness when eating with heartburn.

Some procedures, such as the SG, may exacerbate symptoms of gastroesophageal reflux disease (GERD). Therefore, patients who have moderate to severe GERD may need a conversion to an acid diversion procedure, such as the RYGB. The creation of the small stomach pouch diverts most of the acid produced by the stomach away from the distal esophagus, thus reducing GERD.

Leg Cramps*

Advise patients that cramping with other causes can be managed by doing the following:

- eating a well-balanced diet (include potassium-rich foods, such as yogurt, white beans, tuna, broccoli, cantaloupe, bananas, and milk and magnesium-rich foods, such as nuts and seeds, spinach, avocado, beans, and tofu),
- taking multivitamins and calcium citrate supplements as prescribed daily,
- staying physically active, and
- drinking plenty of fluid.

* Cramping in the legs immediately after surgery can be a sign of a blood clot and is a major medical emergency. Patients should call the medical team immediately if cramps persist or areaccompanied by swelling.

High–Vitamin B12 Levels

If the patient has high levels of vitamin B12 within the first few weeks after surgery, advise the patient to take vitamin B12 one or two times per week instead of daily. Vitamin B12 should continue to be monitored long term, as it can take 3 to 5 years for a vitamin B12 deficiency to develop.[22]

Excessive Hair Shedding and Hair Loss

Hair shedding is normal in the months immediately following MBS, as it is related to rapid weight loss and the acute stress of surgery. It is rarely a sign of a nutritional complication in the immediate postoperative time frame.

Patients may be concerned about hair shedding and hair loss. Advise them about the following:

- Hair shedding is normal in the first few months after surgery and will usually resolve on its own.
- Adequate protein intake and adherence with vitamin and mineral supplements will help prevent hair loss related to nutrient deficiencies.
- In uncomplicated MBS patients, hair shedding in the early postoperative phase is usually related to *telogen effluvium*, not nutritional problems. Studies show an association between low iron and zinc levels and hair loss postoperatively.[23,24] However, it would be naive to recommend special shampoos, extra protein intake, or additional biotin or zinc supplements (beyond the daily multivitamin or dose recommended by the Daily Reference Intakes).

Patients should be assessed for vitamin and mineral deficiencies if hair loss occurs long after the first few postoperative months or if it continues longer than 6 months.

Slow Weight Loss After Metabolic and Bariatric Surgery

Discuss with patients the following reasons they may experience a relatively slow rate of weight loss:

- Most of the immediate rapid weight loss after surgery is loss of excess fluid. Fluid is heavy. Therefore, when the patient is in this phase, the scale shows rapid changes. Once the excess fluid is lost, weight loss will slow down as the patient loses fat, which is lighter than fluid. Body fat takes up space. Therefore, changes in body measurements or changes in how clothes fit more accurately assesses loss of body fat than the scale.
- If the patient lost a significant amount of weight before surgery, they may lose weight slowly after surgery because excess fluid was lost preoperatively.
- If the patient was on a diuretic preoperatively and discontinued it after surgery, loss of excess fluid may take longer. The patient may not lose weight as rapidly as others do.
- If the patient had a lower preoperative body mass index (BMI), they may have less excess fluid to lose following MBS as those with higher BMIs.
- Patients may lose weight slowly if they eat too much because they do not distinguish between physical and emotional hunger or do not recognize physical satiety.
- Some surgeons and MBS providers will prescribe adjuvant weight loss medication in cases of slower weight loss.

Slow Weight Loss After Adjustable Gastric Band

If AGB patients feel that the rate of weight loss within the first few weeks after surgery is too slow, encourage them to do the following:

- Avoid intake of soft high-calorie foods
- Avoid intake of high-calorie beverages
- Avoid drinking with meals
- Understand that weight loss post–adjustable gastric band (AGB) is slower than with other MBS procedures, and patients report more physical hunger after the AGB
- Keep all appointments for band adjustments

Excessive Weight Loss

If the patient's health care team determines that weight loss in the period immediately following MBS is excessive, dehydration may be a cause. Review the patient's food logs to assess food and fluid intake. Consultation with a behavioral therapist is also warranted to assess for changes in mental health status that may impact eating behaviors following surgery. See Chapter 3 for average weight loss rates by procedure type.

References

1. National Institutes of Health Office of Dietary Supplements. Dietary supplement fact sheets: iron. Updated February 28, 2020. Accessed May 31, 2020. http://ods.od.nih.gov/factsheets/Iron-HealthProfessional/#en33
2. van Beek AP, Emous M, Laville M, Tack J. Dumping syndrome after esophageal, gastric or bariatric surgery: pathophysiology, diagnosis, and management. *Obes Rev.* 2017;18(1):68-85. doi:10.1111/obr.12467
3. Tack J, Arts J, Caenepeel P, De Wulf D, Bisschops R. Pathophysiology, diagnosis and management of postoperative dumping syndrome. *Nat Rev Gastroenterol Hepatol.* 2009;6(10):583-590. doi:10.1038/nrgastro.2009.148
4. Ukleja A. Dumping syndrome: pathophysiology and treatment. *Nutr Clin Pr.* 2005;20:517-525. doi:10.1177/0115426505020005517
5. Suhl E, Anderson-Haynes SE, Mulla C, Patti ME. Medical nutrition therapy for post-bariatric hypoglycemia: practical insights. *Surg Obes Relat Dis.* 2017;13(5):888-896. doi:10.1016/j.soard.2017.01.025

6. Carbajo MA, Luque-de-León E, Jiménez JM, Ortiz-de-Solórzano J, Pérez-Miranda M, Castro-Alija MJ. Laparoscopic one-anastomosis gastric bypass: technique, results, and long-term follow-up in 1200 patients. *Obes Surg.* 2017;27(5):1153-1167. doi:10.1007/s11695-016-2428-1
7. Papamargaritis D, Koukoulis G, Sioka E, et al. Dumping symptoms and incidence of hypoglycemia after provocation test at 6 and 12 months after laparoscopic sleeve gastrectomy. *Obes Surg.* 2012;10:1600-1606. doi:10.1007/s11695-012-0711-3
8. Tzovaras G, Papamargaritis D, Sioka E, et al. Symptoms suggestive of dumping syndrome after provocation in patients after laparoscopic sleeve gastrectomy. *Obes Surg.* 2012;22:23-28. doi:10.1007/s11695-011-0461-7
9. Elias K, Bekhali Z, Hedberg J, Graf W, Sundbom M. Changes in bowel habits and patient-scored symptoms after Roux-en-Y gastric bypass and biliopancreatic diversion with duodenal switch. *Surg Obes Relat Dis.* 2018;14(2):144-149. doi:10.1016/j.soard.2017.09.529
10. Solouki A, Kermansaravi M, Davarpanah Jazi AH, Kabir A, Farsani TM, Pazouki A. One-anastomosis gastric bypass as an alternative procedure of choice in morbidly obese patients. *J Res Med Sci.* 2018;23:84. doi:10.4103/jrms.JRMS_386_18
11. Sabate JM, Coupaye M, Ledoux S, et al. Consequences of small intestinal bacterial overgrowth in obese patients before and after bariatric surgery. *Obes Surg.* 2017;27(3):599-605. doi:10.1007/s11695-016-2343-5
12. Sudha MR, Bhonagiri S, Kumar MA. Oral consumption of potential probiotic Saccharomyces boulardii strain Unique 28 in patients with acute diarrhoea: a clinical report. *Benef Microbes.* 2012;3:145-150. doi:10.3920/BM2011.0055
13. Overs SE, Freeman RA, Zarshenas N, Walton KL, Jorgensen JO. Food tolerance and gastrointestinal quality of life following three bariatric procedures: adjustable gastric banding, Roux-en-Y gastric bypass, and sleeve gastrectomy. *Obes Surg.* 2012;22(4):536-543. doi:10.1007/s11695-011-0573-0
14. Allied Health Sciences Section Ad Hoc Nutrition Committee; Aills L, Blankenship J, Buffington C, Furtado M, Parrott J. ASMBS allied health nutritional guidelines for the surgical weight loss patient. *Surg Obes Relat Dis.* 2008;4(5 suppl):S73-S108. doi:10.1016/j.soard.2008.03.002

15. Mechanick JI, Apovian C, Brethauer S, et al. Clinical practice guidelines for the perioperative nutrition, metabolic, and nonsurgical support of patients undergoing bariatric procedures—2019 update: cosponsored by American Association of Clinical Endocrinologists/American College of Endocrinology, the Obesity Society, American Society for Metabolic & Bariatric Surgery, Obesity Medicine Association, and American Society of Anesthesiologists—executive summary. *Endocr Pract.* 2019;25(12):1346-1359. doi:10.4158/GL-2019-0406

16. Mahawar KK, Kumar P, Parmar C, et al. Small bowel limb lengths and Roux-en-Y gastric bypass: a systematic review. *Obes Surg.* 2016;26:660-671. doi:10.1007/s11695-016-2050-2

17. Kuin C, den Ouden F, Brandts H, et al. Treatment of severe protein malnutrition after bariatric surgery. *Obes Surg.* 2019;29(10):3095-3102. doi:10.1007/s11695-019-04035-8

18. Scopinaro N, Marinari GM, Camerini G, et al. Energy and nitrogen absorption after biliopancreatic diversion. *Obes Surg.* 2000;10:436-441. doi:10.1381/096089200321594309

19. Moize V, Geliebter A, Gluck ME, et al. Obese patients have inadequate protein intake related to protein intolerance up to 1 year following Roux-en-Y gastric bypass. *Obes Surg.* 2003;13(1):23-28. doi:10.1381/096089203321136548

20. Skroubis G, Sakellaropoulos G, Pouggouras K, Mead N, Nikiforidis G, Kalfarentzos F. Comparison of nutritional deficiencies after Roux-en-Y gastric bypass and after biliopancreatic diversion with Roux-en-Y gastric bypass. *Obes Surg.* 2002;12(4):551-558. doi:10.1381/096089202762252334

21. Skroubis G, Anesidis S, Kehagias I, Mead N, Vagenas K, Kalfarentzos F. Roux-en-Y gastric bypass versus a variant of biliopancreatic diversion in a non-superobese population: prospective comparison of the efficacy and the incidence of metabolic deficiencies. *Obes Surg.* 2006;16(4):488-495. doi:10.1381/096089206776327251

22. Johnson LE. Vitamin B12 deficiency. Merck Manual. October 2019. Accessed August 1, 2020. www.merckmanuals.com/home/disorders-of-nutrition/vitamins/vitamin-b12-deficiency#:~:text=Unlike%20most%20other%20vitamins%2C%20B12,to%205%20years%20to%20exhaust

23. Ruiz-Tovar J, Oller I, Llavero C, et al. Hair loss in females after sleeve gastrectomy: predictive value of serum zinc and iron levels. *Am Surg.* 2014;80(5):466-471.

24. Katsogridaki G, Tzovaras G, Sioka E, et al. Hair loss after laparoscopic sleeve gastrectomy. *Obes Surg.* 2018;28:3929-3934. doi:10.1007/s11695-018-3433-3

APPENDIX H

Nutrition Counseling and Education

Like with any type of patient interaction, providing facts and diets is not effective without techniques to encourage behavior change. Counseling strategies and theoretical models from food-related research and social psychology are used to guide nutrition interventions.[1] Components of cognitive and behavioral therapies are also used to promote goal setting and behavior modification. There are many tools available for the registered dietitian nutritionist (RDN) working with metabolic and bariatric surgery (MBS) patients to help them implement short-term and long-term diet and lifestyle changes after surgery.

Behavior Change

The goals of nutrition counseling are to facilitate lifestyle awareness, to reinforce good decision-making, and to learn how to take appropriate action.[1] This means the RDN plays a critical role in helping MBS patients implement behavior change. Behavior change can be challenging because it means the patient must conduct themselves differently in some particular manner. The longer the old behavior has been followed, the harder it is to change. Behavior change models, such as the health belief model or the transtheoretical model (TTM), provide insight into the patient's individual factors (eg, knowledge, attitudes, beliefs, prior experiences) that may affect their ability to change. There are many counseling tools available to RDNs to assist their MBS patients in behavior change. Cognitive behavioral therapy (CBT) has been shown to be effective for changing health behaviors, and motivational interviewing (MI) has been especially helpful in working with patients who are in the early stages of behavior change.

Health Belief Model

The health belief model poses that cognitive factors influence an individual's decision to make and maintain a specific health behavior change.[2] An individual's ability to make a decision related to their health behavior depends on (1) their perceived personal susceptibility to a disease of condition, (2) their perception of the disease or condition as having some degree of severity, (3) their belief that there are particular benefits in taking actions that would help the disease or condition, (4) their perception that no major barriers would prevent the health action, (5) their exposure to a stimulus to take action, and (6) their confidence in their ability to implement the behavior (ie, self-efficacy).[1] All of these beliefs interact with each other to prompt a patient's willingness to make a change.

An MBS patient's motivation to make changes in their eating habits after surgery will depend on the severity of their comorbidities and their perception of the severity of the disease to their overall health. The fact that a patient has decided to undergo MBS surgery is evidence of their belief that their health is under threat. In addition, the consequences of their health condition may prompt them to make a change. For example, a patient may be motivated to change due to fear of taking insulin for their type 2 diabetes when their hemoglobin A1c is elevated. The RDN can better work with each MBS patient by understanding what they perceive within each health belief construct. Asking the patient their goal of surgery or goal of a particular counseling session can help align the patient's perspective and the RDN's agenda.

The Transtheoretical Model (Stages of Change)

TTM is also known as the stages of change; it was developed by Prochaska and DiClemente. It incorporates many psychotherapy and counseling theories. Each stage is known as a motivational stage and includes the following: (1) precontemplation, (2) contemplation, (3) preparation, (4) action, (5) maintenance, and (6) termination.[1] Patients will have different nutritional and behavioral strategies that work for them at different stages. In working with MBS patients, RDNs can stay alert to key words and behaviors that indicate in which stage the patient falls for making a behavior change. For example, the MBS patient who says they won't stop eating foods containing high amounts of added sugar is in the precontemplation stage. They will not be persuaded to change this behavior by threat or force. The patient needs to hear that making the change is their choice, but they could benefit from hearing about the personalized benefits of changing and the ways the changes could be made.

Cognitive Behavioral Therapy

Cognitive behavioral therapy (CBT) includes components of cognitive therapies and behavior therapy. It includes a wide range of treatment approaches.[1] The Academy of Nutrition and Dietetics expert panel analysis considers CBT to be a highly effective form of nutrition counseling theoretical approach for changing health and food behavior.[3] Common approaches to using behavior modification include the following: (1) classical conditioning, (2) operant conditioning, and (3) modeling.

Classical conditioning uses stimuli or cues that affect food behavior.[1] In working with MBS patients, RDNs may encourage patients to eliminate foods from their homes that are difficult to eat or tolerate during their early postoperative period, such as beef, sweets, juice, soft bread, pasta, and rice, so that patients are not tempted to consume them and feel they are depriving themselves of those items. Operant conditioning is based on the idea that behaviors can be changed for a positive of negative effect.[4,5] For example, RDNs might encourage MBS patients to treat themselves to a nonfood reward when they avoid a triggering food or meet a particular health goal. Lastly, modeling is provided to the MBS patient via cooking demonstrations, support groups, and observational learning.

Motivational Interviewing

This approach to counseling integrates client-centered counseling and the TTM. It focuses on strategies to help motivate patients to make a behavior change and commit to it.[6] MI helps to identify the patient's natural motivation for change (intrinsic motivation). Patients can have intrinsic or extrinsic (those coerced by external forces) motivation as a result of their values.[1] This allows for enhanced performance, persistence, and creativity to accomplish the task of behavior change. Since MBS RDNs can impact motivation, it is considered an essential part of their nutrition intervention.

The spirit of MI reminds the RDN to resist the righting reflex.[6] RDNs want to see their patients succeed. If a patient is ambivalent to change or has a good argument for not changing, the RDN may be prompted to set things straight and confirm the correct reasons for changing a food behavior. For example, a new MBS patient who avoids fruit may think that they must do so in order to avoid sugar and prevent dumping syndrome. Although it is appropriate to inform the patient that fruit contains natural sugar that would not lead to dumping syndrome, the patient may have already made up their mind that they must avoid fruit, and so attempts to change their mind will be futile. Not until the MBS patient and RDN form a partnership, interact with the understanding of acceptance and compassion, as well as the assumption of evocation, will the spirit of MI be incorporated into the RDNs counseling techniques.

Implementing Motivational Interviewing With Other Behavior Change Approaches

It is important to note that MI is not the only counseling strategy that can be provided by the RDN. MI can be utilized with CBT, goal setting, solution-focused therapy, the concept of self-efficacy, and other counseling techniques to support the patient in making a behavior change. Identification of the appropriate technique requires the clinical discretion of the RDN.

Solution-Focused Therapy

Solution-focused therapists work with patients to identify solutions that have worked for them in the past and expand on them.[1] The focus of sessions is on the one time the patient's actions worked. Despite the name, solution-focused therapy does not focus on solving problems. For example, an adolescent MBS patient complains that their parents keep junk food snacks in the house, causing an ongoing challenge. They would be asked to think of a time when they avoided those snacks or chose a healthy snack of their own instead of those of their parents.

Client-Centered Counseling

Also known as person-centered counseling, the basic foundation of this theory of counseling is that human beings are rational, socialized, and realistic. They have an inherent tendency to strive toward growth, self-actualization, and self-direction.[1] Therefore, it is not the RDN's job to tell the patient what to do. RDNs can develop a patient-centered environment by not passing judgment on their patients' thoughts, behaviors, or physiques. This means the RDN must set aside their own beliefs and respect their patient, regardless of whether they have followed medical and counseling advice.

RDNs working with MBS patients can demonstrate client-centered therapy with verbal and nonverbal acceptance, empathy, and support that acknowledges the challenges of making changes before and after MBS surgery. The RDN also supports the patient when they meet a barrier to those changes.

Shared Decision-Making

The principles of shared decision-making strengthen the principles of patient-centered care. It is a communication process in which the patient and RDN work together to make decisions that are best for the patient. Shared decision-making promotes self-determination and supports autonomy throughout the relationship.[7] The RDN must communicate with the patient to determine what is most important to them before recommending they make a behavior change. Shared decision-making could be utilized when working toward choosing a multivitamin and supplement regimen; the RDN chooses the supplements based on their clinical knowledge and matches it with the patient's preferences for cost, delivery method, options for purchasing, number of pills, and so on.

Empathy

The relationship between the MBS patient and the RDN relies on the RDN's ability to experience and show empathy. A relationship will not move forward without empathy. Patient outcomes have been shown to be affected by the counselor's degree of empathy.[8]

Cultural Influences

Verbal and nonverbal behavior will differ based on the cultural orientation of the patient and the RDN. Culture influences communication and the closer the two individuals share a common culture, the greater the likelihood that misperceptions will be minimized.[1] Individual variation exists within any particular cultural group, but RDNs must be aware of different communication styles and recognize in which culture they are practicing. More importantly, the RDN must craft their counseling style and nutrition recommendations to the patient's needs. These needs include the patient's culture. Telling a patient to stop eating their cultural foods is ineffective and naive.

Nutrition Education

The Academy of Nutrition and Dietetics defines nutrition education as "reinforcement of basic or essential nutrition-related knowledge."[9] Nutrition counseling differs from nutrition education, but nutrition education is a primary step to change diet behavior.[10] Effective nutrition education language avoids the use of commands and supports a desire to make changes. RDNs use supportive language and avoid using the phrase, "you should."[5] For example, the RDN might say, "I hear you. You are frustrated with feeling lightheaded and fatigued after eating. I have a few suggestions that I believe will help you feel better after eating. Would you like to hear them?"

Conclusion

The RDN can successfully form a long-term working relationship with the MBS patient by implementing a variety of counseling techniques and understanding psychological theories of behavior change. The patient may have had previous experiences with bias in the medical field, so reestablishing a supportive relationship of empathy, understanding, and a safe place of nonjudgment can both help the patient reach their goals and also reestablish trust for the role of the RDN and medical professionals.

References

1. Bauer KD, Liou D. *Nutrition Counseling and Education Skill Development*. 4th ed. Cengage; 2021.
2. Rosenstock M, Strecher VJ, Becker mg. Social learning theory and the health belief model. *Health Educ Quart*. 1988;15:175-183. doi:10.1177/109019818801500203
3. Spahn JM, Reeves RS, Keim KS, et al. State of the evidence regarding behavior change theories and strategies in nutrition counseling to facilitate health and food-behavior change. *J Am Diet Assoc*. 2010;110:879-891. doi:10.1016/j.jada.2010.03.021

4. Kellogg M. *Counseling Tips for Nutrition Therapists, Practice Workbook*. Vol 1. Kg Press; 2006.
5. Kellogg M. *Counseling Tips for Nutrition Therapists, Practice Workbook*. Vol 2. Kg Press; 2009.
6. Rollnick S, Miller W. *Motivational Interviewing: Helping People Change*. 3rd ed. Guilford Press; 2012.
7. Elwyn G, Frosch D, Thomson R, et al. Shared decision making: a model for clinical practice. *J Gen Intern Med*. 2012;27(10):1361-1367. doi:10.1007/s11606-012-2077-6
8. Rollnick P, Mason P, Butler C. *Health Behavior Change: A Guide for Practitioners*. Churchill Livingstone; 1999.
9. Academy of Nutrition and Dietetics. MNT versus Nutrition Education. Academy of Nutrition and Dietetics. August 2006. Accessed January 9, 2021. https:/eatrightpro.org/payment/coding-and-billing/mnt-vs-nutrition-education
10. Brownell KD, Cohen R. Adherence to dietary regimens. 2: components of effective intervention. *Behav Med*. 1995;20(4):155-164. doi:10.1080/08964289.1995.9933732

Continuing Professional Education

The third edition of the *Academy of Nutrition and Dietetics Pocket Guide to Bariatric Surgery* offers readers 7 hours of Continuing Professional Education (CPE) credit. Readers may earn credit by completing the interactive quiz at:

https://publications.webauthor.com/pg_bariatric_3rd_ed

Index